Diagnosis and Management of Bowel Diseases

Second Edition

Paul F. Engstrom, MD

Professor of Medicine
Temple University School of Medicine
Adjunct Professor of Medicine
University of Pennsylvania School of Medicine
Senior Vice President for Population Science
Fox Chase Cancer Center
Philadelphia, PA

Eric B. Goosenberg, MD

Assistant Professor of Medicine
Temple University School of Medicine
Attending Gastroenterologist
Abington Memorial Hospital, Abington, PA
Holy Redeemer Hospital, Meadowbrook, PA

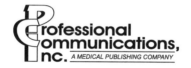

Professional Communications, Inc.
A MEDICAL PUBLISHING COMPANY

Published by
Professional Communications, Inc.

Marketing Office:
400 Center Bay Drive
West Islip, NY 11795
(t) 631/661-2852
(f) 631/661-2167

Editorial Office:
PO Box 10
Caddo, OK 74729-0010
(t) 580/367-9838
(f) 580/367-9989

For orders only, please call
1-800-337-9838

or visit our website at
www.pcibooks.com

ISBN: 1-884735-88-6

Printed in the United States of America

DISCLAIMER
The opinions expressed in this publication reflect those of the authors. However, the authors make no warranty regarding the contents of the publication. The protocols described herein are general and may not apply to a specific patient. Any product mentioned in this publication should be taken in accordance with the prescribing information provided by the manufacturer.

This text is printed on recycled paper.

DEDICATION

*To my beautiful family who graciously gave
me the time I needed to prepare this book:
my wife, Robyn,
and my children,
Scott, Hallie, and David.*
—**EBG**

*To Dr. Maria Engstrom Pharr
for continuing the family medical tradition;
may she and other primary-care physicians
benefit from this handbook.*
—**PFE**

ACKNOWLEDGMENT

The authors would like to express their thanks to Malcolm Beasley and Phyllis Jones Freeny at Professional Communications, Inc. for their assistance and efforts in the preparation of this manuscript and to Nikki D. Merrill for her graphic design work.

I would like to thank Drs. Deren, Bralow, Retig, Greenfield, and Ahtaridis, whose enouragement and skills prepared me so well to enter the field of gastroenterology. Thanks also to my colleagues, Stuart Lubinski, MD and Robert Stein, MD, for their input and advice in updates to the text.

—**EBG**

I would like to thank Marion Keefe for typing the manuscript and corresponding with the publisher.

—**PFE**

TABLE OF CONTENTS

TABLES

FIGURES

ix

Introduction

This handbook was written for students and practitioners who evaluate and treat maladies of the gastrointestinal (GI) tract. Diarrhea, as well as a number of relatively common benign and malignant conditions that cause lower GI symptoms, is reviewed in detail, with published practice guidelines applied when available. Clinical research is on the cusp of major advances in the understanding of the genetics and medical management of at least two of the illnesses discussed herein, inflammatory bowel disease and colorectal cancer. Hopefully, future publications will paint a somewhat rosier picture for those afflicted with these very serious conditions, and a great deal of effort is being expended toward this end.

Diarrhea is discussed in terms of the various pathophysiologic mechanisms responsible, with a differential diagnosis and clinical approach presented based on a number of relatively frequently encountered clinical settings. Practice parameters published by the American College of Gastroenterology are used to guide the reader through management decision-making in acute infectious diarrhea.

Irritable bowel syndrome is likely to be managed more effectively in the future by an increased familiarity with the use of low-dose antidepressant medications as well as hormonal therapy. Recognition that this condition may also cause a wide variety of clinical manifestations, particularly psychological, is critical to an appreciation of the importance of the physician-patient relationship in the management of this extremely common problem.

Diverticular disease of the colon may become less common in the future with more attention toward greater fiber intake by Americans, but it is currently seen quite frequently in clinical practice, usually as a cause of abdominal pain or lower GI bleeding. The use of percutaneous drainage of abscesses or collections in acute diverticulitis offers the benefit of reducing what has often been a two-step surgical procedure into a single, open operation in many patients.

Inflammatory bowel disease, comprised of ulcerative colitis and Crohn's disease, has been the subject of intense clinical research in recent years due in large part to the efforts of a number of supportive organizations, including the Crohn's and Colitis Foundation of America and its counterparts elsewhere around the world. Practice guidelines for these conditions, also published by the American College of Gastroenterology, are provided; however, with the addition of newer agents such as immunomodulators, cytokines, and monoclonal antibodies into the treatment armamentarium, such guidelines will likely remain in flux for the next several years.

The chapter on colorectal cancer emphasizes pathogenesis, screening, diagnosis, and management of the disease. Scientific discovery in molecular genetics, chemoprevention, and cancer chemotherapy is likely to greatly impact how physicians manage patients at risk for colon cancer and those who have potentially curable disease. Future editions of this handbook are likely to address the use of molecular probes to screen the stool for genetic markers of cancer, to emphasize mutation analysis in high-risk family members, to discuss proven prevention interventions and to feature combination cancer therapy using cell-signal transmitters in conjunction with anticancer drugs.

1 Diarrhea: General Information

Diarrhea is a term used for:
- Either loose or watery stools
- Excessive or increased stool frequency
- An excessive volume of stool passed.

The first of these descriptions is most suggestive of pathology. The frequency of bowel movements and volume of stool can vary significantly from individual to individual without necessarily being sensed subjectively as diarrhea. Normal daily stool volume is <200 g, but frequent small stools may not exceed this volume, and larger volumes of solid stool are not necessarily pathologic.

Persons at highest risk of developing diarrhea include:
- Those exposed to contaminated food or water
- Those in close contact with infants and children (eg, in day-care centers)
- World travelers
- Homosexual males
- Those who are immunocompromised.

Diarrhea is usually due to one of four pathophysiologic mechanisms (although more than one mechanism may be in effect in an individual patient):
- Osmotic diarrhea: due to excessive ingestion of poorly absorbable osmotically active solutes in the intestinal lumen (**Table 1.1**)
- Secretory diarrhea: due to either excessive intestinal ion secretion or inadequate ion absorption (**Table 1.2**)

TABLE 1.1 — CAUSES OF OSMOTIC DIARRHEA

Carbohydrate Malabsorption
- Congenital glucose-galactose malabsorption
- Congenital fructose malabsorption
- Disaccharidase deficiencies (congenital or acquired):
  - Lactase deficiency
  - Sucrase-isomaltose deficiency (causing diarrhea from sorbitol ingestion)
- Generalized malabsorption syndrome
- Excessive ingestion of poorly absorbable carbohydrate:
  - Lactulose
  - Sorbitol and mannitol (elixirs, sugar-free gum or mints, fruit)
  - Fructose (fruits, soft drinks)
  - Fiber (bran, fruits, vegetables)

Magnesium-Induced Diarrhea
- Nutrition supplements
- Antacids
- Laxatives

Gastrointestinal Lavage Solutions Containing Polyethylene Glycol (PEG)
- GoLYTELY
- CoLYTE
- NuLYTELY

Laxatives Containing Sodium and a Poorly Absorbable Anion
- Sodium citrate
- Sodium phosphate
- Sodium sulfate

- Intestinal dysmotility (**Table 1.3**)
- Exudative or inflammatory diarrhea: due to passage of blood, mucus, or protein in the stool (**Table 1.4**).

Approach to the Patient With Diarrhea

■ Clinical History

The patient's description of symptoms often provides clues that may help to determine the underlying cause of diarrhea (**Table 1.5**).

■ Physical Examination

In acute diarrhea, the examination is more useful as a marker of severity of disease (eg, fever, lymphadenopathy, or signs of dehydration) than in reaching a specific diagnosis. A number of physical findings may be helpful in diagnosing the etiology of chronic diarrhea (**Table 1.6**).

SUGGESTED READING

McCray WH, Krevsky B. Diagnosing diarrhea in adults: a practical approach. *Hosp Med.* 1998;34:27-36.

TABLE 1.2 — CONDITIONS ASSOCIATED WITH SECRETORY DIARRHEA

Infections
- Enterotoxigenic bacteria
- Chronic mycobacterial, fungal, or parasitic infections

Stimulant Laxatives
- Ricinoleic acid
- Phenolphthalein
- Bisacodyl
- Docusate sodium
- Cascara
- Aloe
- Senna
- Danthron

Intestinal Resection

Inflammatory Bowel Diseases
- Ulcerative colitis
- Crohn's disease
- Microscopic (collagenous and lymphocytic) colitis

Bile Acid Malabsorption
- Terminal ileal disease, bypass, or resection
- After truncal vagotomy and cholecystectomy
- Idiopathic, due to abnormal ileal transport of bile acids

Fatty Acid Malabsorption
- Chronic cholestasis (eg, primary biliary cirrhosis)
- Pancreatic insufficiency

Malabsorption due to:
- Small intestinal disease:
  - Celiac and tropical sprue
  - Lymphangiectasia
  - Inflammatory bowel disease
  - Abetalipoproteinemia
  - Giardiasis or cryptosporidiosis
  - Lymphoma

- Anatomic changes:
  - Surgical small-bowel bypass (eg, jejunoileal bypass)
  - Short bowel syndrome
  - Postgastrectomy/postvagotomy ("dumping syndrome")
  - Fistulas from the luminal gastrointestinal tract
- Maldigestion due to pancreatic insufficiency, bacterial overgrowth, or biliary obstruction

Benign or Malignant Tumors
- Rectal villous adenomas
- Lymphoma of the small bowel
- Zollinger-Ellison syndrome
- Pancreatic cholera (VIP-oma) causing WDHA
- Malignant carcinoid syndrome
- Medullary carcinoma of the thyroid
- Glucagonoma

Collagen Vascular Diseases
- Systemic lupus erythematosus
- Progressive systemic sclerosis (scleroderma)
- Mixed connective tissue disease

Abbreviations: VIP, vasoactive intestinal peptide; WDHA, watery diarrhea, hypokalemia, achlorhydria.

TABLE 1.3 — DIARRHEA DUE TO DYSMOTILITY

- Irritable bowel syndrome (IBS)
- Fecal impaction and incontinence
- Diabetes mellitus
- Scleroderma
- Hyperthyroidism
- Drug side effect
- Adhesive chronic partial bowel obstruction
- Intestinal blind loop syndrome

TABLE 1.4 — EXUDATIVE OR INFLAMMATORY DIARRHEA

- Infectious diarrhea
- Neoplastic disease (lymphoma, carcinoma)
- Radiation enteritis or colitis
- Chemotherapy-induced enteritis or colitis
- Inflammatory bowel disease
- Ischemic colitis

TABLE 1.5 — CLUES TO DIAGNOSIS OF DIARRHEA BASED ON ASSOCIATED SYMPTOMS

Symptoms Associated With Diarrhea	Relevant Diagnoses
Bloody stools	Inflammatory, infectious or neoplastic conditions
Alternating constipation and diarrhea	Irritable bowel syndrome (IBS), diabetic autonomic neuropathy, intermittent bowel obstruction, patients who are intermittently medicating themselves for either constipation or diarrhea
Oily or greasy stools	Fat malabsorption (particularly pancreatic insufficiency)
Large volume diarrhea	Disease involving the small bowel or proximal colon
Small volume diarrhea	Rectal or distal colonic disease
Diarrhea with excessive flatus	Carbohydrate malabsorption
Family history of diarrhea	Inflammatory bowel disease (IBD), congenital absorption defect, celiac sprue
Recent antibiotic exposure	*Clostridium difficile* colitis
Recent travel to a mountainous area	*Giardia* infestation
Fever	IBD, lymphoma, Whipple's disease, hyperthyroidism, many infectious diseases
Weight loss	Malabsorption, IBD, malignancy
Work in a day-care center for children	Infection with *Shigella* species, *Giardia lamblia*, or *Cryptosporidium*
Flushing	Hyperthyroidism, carcinoid syndrome, pheochromocytoma, pancreatic cholera, systemic mastocytosis

TABLE 1.6 — CLUES TO DIAGNOSIS OF DIARRHEA BASED ON PHYSICAL FINDINGS

Physical Finding Associated With Diarrhea	Relevant Diagnoses
Oral ulcers	Inflammatory bowel disease (IBD), celiac sprue
Arthritis	IBD, Whipple's disease, enteritis due to infection with *Salmonella, Shigella, Yersinia* and *Campylobacter* species, collagen vascular disease, collagenous colitis, gonococcal proctitis
Systemic atherosclerosis	Mesenteric ischemia, ischemic colitis
Lymphadenopathy	Small bowel lymphoma, Whipple's disease, acquired immunodeficiency syndrome, metastatic cancer
Neuropathy	Diabetes mellitus, amyloidosis
Postural hypotension	Diabetic diarrhea, Addison's disease
Cutaneous erythema	Glucagonoma syndrome, systemic mastocytosis
Cutaneous hyperpigmentation	Whipple's disease, sprue, Addison's disease, systemic mastocytosis
Dermatitis herpetiformis	Celiac sprue
Pyoderma gangrenosum	IBD

2

Diarrhea: Acute Diarrhea and Diarrhea in AIDS

Acute diarrhea (lasting less than 3 weeks) is most often due to viruses, bacteria, food poisoning, or drugs (**Table 2.1**). Although infections are the most common etiology, alcohol excess, food intolerance, and drug side effects should always be considered. If diarrhea begins soon after beginning a new medication, thought should be given to discontinuing the medication on a trial basis, even if diarrhea is not reported as a common side effect.

Acute infectious diarrhea is often mild and self-limited, and extensive stool studies are typically unnecessary. Evaluation of acute diarrhea for a specific pathogen should be carried out only under the following conditions:

- Dehydration or clinical toxicity
- Immunocompromised patient
- Bloody stools (in the absence of an unrelated anorectal cause such as internal hemorrhoids or an anal fissure)
- Persistence or worsening of symptoms over more than 5 to 7 days.

Recipients of anal intercourse (homosexual males and some women) are prone to certain infectious causes of diarrhea that are not seen in other populations, including:

- Proctitis due to gonorrhea
- *Chlamydia trachomatis*
- Herpes simplex
- Syphilis
- *Entamoeba histolytica.*

TABLE 2.1 — MAJOR CAUSES OF ACUTE DIARRHEA

Infections
- Bacterial (including traveler's diarrhea):
  - *Campylobacter* species
  - *Clostridium difficile*
  - *Escherichia coli* (enterotoxigenic, enteroinvasive, enterohemorrhagic, and 0157:H7)
  - *Salmonella enteritidis*
  - *Shigella* species
  - *Yersinia*
  - *Aeromonas*
- Parasitic/protozoal:
  - *Entamoeba histolytica*
  - *Giardia lamblia*
  - *Cryptosporidium*
  - *Cyclospora*
- Viral:
  - Adenovirus
  - Norwalk virus
  - Rotavirus
  - Others

Food Poisoning
- *Bacillus cereus*
- *Clostridium perfringens*
- *Salmonella* species
- *Staphylococcus aureus*
- *Vibrio* species
- *Shigella* species
- *Campylobacter jejuni*
- *Escherichia coli*
- *Yersinia enterocolitica*
- *Listeria monocytogenes*

Medications
- Antibiotics:
  - Side effects
  - Antibiotic-induced diarrhea due to *Clostridium difficile*, *Clostridium perfringens*, *Salmonella* species, and, possibly, *Candida albicans*

- Chemotherapy (eg, methotrexate, 5-fluorouracil)
- Colchicine
- Digoxin
- Diuretics
- Histamine-2 receptor antagonists
- Lactose or sorbitol in elixir medications
- Laxatives
- Magnesium-containing drugs
- Nonsteroidal anti-inflammatory drugs
- Quinidine

Miscellaneous
- Recent ingestion of large amount of poorly absorbable sugars
- Intestinal ischemia
- Fecal impaction
- Pelvic inflammation
- Therapeutic radiation (for endometrial, cervical, prostate, or rectal cancer)

Patients with acquired immunodeficiency disease (AIDS) and those in other immunodeficient states are at risk for a number of opportunistic infections that may cause diarrhea and significant debility (**Table 2.2**).

Traveler's Diarrhea

Risk of developing traveler's diarrhea approaches 40% when traveling to high-risk areas of the world (such as to southern Asia, northern Africa, Central and South America). Most cases of endemic diarrhea are due to pathogenic bacteria, though viruses and parasitic infections are also relatively frequent. Infections causing traveler's diarrhea include:
- Bacteria:
  - *Shigella* species
  - *Salmonella* species
  - *Yersinia enterocolitica*
  - *Aeromonas* species
  - Enterotoxigenic *Escherichia coli* (ETEC)

TABLE 2.2 — DIFFERENTIAL DIAGNOSIS OF DIARRHEA IN AIDS

Bacteria
- *Salmonella* species*
- *Shigella* species*
- *Campylobacter* species*
- *Mycobacterium avium* complex (MAC)
- *Chlamydia trachomatis*
- *Clostridium difficile*
- *Vibrio* species
- Small bowel bacterial overgrowth

Protozoa
- *Cryptosporidium**
- Microsporidia*
- *Cyclospora cayatanensis*
- *Entamoeba histolytica*
- *Giardia lamblia*
- *Isospora belli*
- *Leishmania donovani*
- *Blastocystis hominis*
- *Pneumocystis carinii*

Viruses
- Cytomegalovirus* (CMV)
- Herpes simplex
- Adenovirus
- Rotavirus
- Norwalk virus
- Human immunodeficiency virus (HIV) (controversial)

Fungi
- *Histoplasma* species
- *Coccidioides*
- *Candida albicans*
- *Cryptococcus*

Intestinal Tumors
- Lymphoma
- Kaposi's sarcoma

2

  - *Staphylococcus aureus*
  - *Bacillus cereus*
  - *Clostridium difficile*
  - *Listeria monocytogenes*
  - Rotavirus
  - Norwalk virus
- Parasites:
  - *Giardia lamblia*
  - *Entamoeba histolytica.*

Prophylactic antibiotics are not recommended in general, but if necessary, treatment can be given for the first 2 weeks of travel with bismuth subsalicylate (Pepto-Bismol) two tablets po qid or ciprofloxacin 500 mg/day. Prophylactic therapy is suggested for people with the following underlying conditions:
- AIDS
- Inflammatory bowel disease
- Prior gastric surgery or use of proton pump inhibitor medication (omeprazole, lansoprazole, rabeprazole, pantoprazole, or esomeprazole), which may result in hypochlorhydria
- Insulin-dependent diabetes mellitus

- Malignancy
- An inability to tolerate a brief illness while traveling.

All travelers to high-risk regions should take loperamide and antibiotics with them to treat themselves if necessary. Treatment should be initiated as soon as diarrhea begins. Therapeutic options include:
- Loperamide (Imodium) 4 mg initially, then 2 mg after each loose stool (to a maximum of 16 mg/day) plus any one of the following three fluoroquinolones, all taken orally for 3 days:
  - Ciprofloxacin 500 mg po bid
  - Levofloxacin 500 mg po daily
  - Ofloxacin 300 mg bid
- Loperamide with azithromycin (500 mg po initially, then 250 mg po daily for 4 days, or 1000 mg po for one dose) if fluoroquinolones cannot be used.

Empiric Treatment in Acute Infectious Diarrhea

Empiric antimicrobial therapy without a formal evaluation should be considered in patients of two types:
- Those in whom bacterial diarrhea is likely, based on clinical features or on leukocytes or blood in the stool
- Patients whose diarrhea has persisted for more than 2 weeks and in whom infection with *Giardia* is strongly suspected.

Other indications for treatment of acute diarrhea are shown in **Table 2.3**.

TABLE 2.3 — INDICATIONS FOR EMPIRIC AND SPECIFIC ANTIMICROBIAL THERAPY IN INFECTIOUS DIARRHEA

Indication for Antimicrobial Therapy	Suggested Therapy
Fever plus one of the following: • Dysentery (grossly bloody stools) • Leukocyte-, lactoferrin- or Hemoccult-positive stools	Fluoroquinolones: ciprofloxacin 500 mg or ofloxacin 300 mg bid for 3 days, or levofloxacin 500 mg once daily for 3 days
Moderate to severe traveler's diarrhea	The fluoroquinolones at above dosages for 1 to 5 days
Persistent diarrhea (*Giardia* suspected)	Metronidazole 250 mg qid for 7 days
Shigella infection	If acquired in the United States, give ciprofloxacin 500 mg or ofloxacin 300 mg bid for 3 days, trimethoprim/sulfamethoxazole (TMP/SMX) 160/800 mg bid for 3 days, or azithromycin 500 mg po initially, then 250 mg po daily for 4 days; if during international travel, treat as febrile dysentery (as above); be sure to check for drug sensitivity of organism
Salmonella infection	If healthy host with mild to moderate symptoms, no treatment is needed. If severe illness with fever and clinical toxicity or if an underlying condition increases risk of bacteremia (see text) use ciprofloxacin 500 mg bid for 5 to 7 days or azithromycin 1 g po once, then 500 mg po daily for 6 days

Continued

Indication for Antimicrobial Therapy	Suggested Therapy
Campylobacter jejuni infection	Azithromycin 500 mg po daily or ciprofloxacin 500 mg po bid for 3 days; alternatively, erythromycin stearate 500 mg po qid for 5 days can be used
Escherichia coli	
• Enteropathogenic (EPEC)	Treat as febrile dysentery
• Enterotoxigenic (ETEC)	Treat as moderate to severe traveler's diarrhea
• Enteroinvasive (EIEC)	Treat as shigellosis
• Enterohemorrhagic (EHEC or *E. coli* 0157:H7)	Antimicrobials should not be given
Aeromonas diarrhea	Treat as febrile dysentery
Vibrio cholerae	Ciprofloxacin 1 g po or doxycycline 300 mg po for 1 dose; hydration is the most important treatment, either IV (4 g NaCl + 1 g KCl + 5.4 g Na lactate + 8 g glucose per liter) or po (1 level teaspoon of table salt + 4 heaping teaspoons of sugar per liter), replacing the volume lost[1]
Noncholera *Vibrio* diarrhea	Treat as febrile dysentery

Yersinia infection	For most cases, treat as for *Shigella*; for severe cases, give ceftriaxone 2 g IV daily for 5 days
Giardiasis	Metronidazole 250 mg tid for 5 days or furazolidone 100 mg po qid for 7 to 10 days
Intestinal amebiasis	Metronidazole 500-750 mg tid for 10 days then a drug to treat cysts to prevent relapses: • Iodoquinol 650 mg tid for 20 days, or • Paromomycin 500 mg tid for 7 days
Cryptosporidium diarrhea	Hydration only in immunocompetent patients
Isospora diarrhea	TMP/SMX 160/800 mg bid for 10 days in immunocompetent patients
Cyclospora diarrhea	TMP/SMX 160/800 mg bid for 7 days

[1] Reference: Levine MM, et al. *J Trop Med Hyg.* 1981;84:73-76.

Adapted from: DuPont HL. *Am J Gastroenterol.* 1997;92:1962-1975; *The Sanford Guide to Antimicrobial Therapy,* 2003.

Foodborne or Waterborne Outbreaks of Diarrhea

An epidemic of diarrhea after a social gathering suggests food poisoning. When fever and/or dysentery (many small-volume stools containing blood and mucus) are experienced in most of the affected individuals, a number of organisms may be responsible. They include the invasive bacterial pathogens (*Shigella, Salmonella,* or *Campylobacter* species) or other pathogens that clinically simulate them, such as enteroinvasive *E coli, Aeromonas* species, and noncholera *Vibrio* bacteria. The time between the ingestion and onset of symptoms (the incubation period) may be helpful in identifying possible infectious culprits (**Table 2.4**).

TABLE 2.4 — RELATIONSHIP OF TIME AND ORGANISMS CAUSING FOODBORNE DIARRHEAL OUTBREAKS

Incubation Period	Organisms Possibly Responsible
Within 6 hours	*Staphylococcus aureus, Bacillus cereus*
8 to 14 hours	*Clostridium perfringens*
>14 hours (especially if vomiting predominates over diarrhea)	Enteric viruses

Evaluation of the Patient With Acute Diarrhea

If acute infectious diarrhea is suspected, the Practice Parameters Committee of the American College of Gastroenterology recommends that medical evaluation be limited to patients who are more severely ill or those whose history suggests a specific pathogen. In most other circumstances, the diarrhea is likely to be self-limited and need not be treated or evaluated for a specific pathogen. Indications for evaluation include:

- Profuse diarrhea with dehydration
- Dysentery
- High fever (oral temperature of at least 101.3°F or 38.5°C) suggests invasive bacteria (*Shigella*, *Salmonella*, or *Campylobacter* species) an enteric virus, or a cytotoxic organism damaging the mucosa such as *C difficile* or *E histolytica*
- More than 6 stools in a 24-hour period or duration of illness longer than 2 days, since patients with this degree of illness may benefit from empiric therapy
- Diarrhea with severe abdominal pain in a patient >50 years of age, to evaluate for ischemic disease
- Diarrhea in the elderly (≥70 years of age), in whom severe or prolonged diarrhea is potentially fatal
- Immunocompromised patients (those with AIDS, those who have received an organ transplant, or patients who are receiving cancer chemotherapy)
- Patients with diarrhea lasting 2 to 4 weeks who do not have dysentery or systemic symptoms; such individuals should either undergo diagnostic evaluation or be treated empirically for giardiasis (**Table 2.3**). Stool studies are frequently negative for *Giardia* protozoa when this organism is responsible for clinical illness, so a workup in this clinical setting might best be reserved for patients who fail to respond to an empiric course of metronidazole.

Recommended laboratory testing includes:

- Stool testing for occult blood, leukocytes, and possibly for lactoferrin
- A stool culture (for *Salmonella*, *Shigella*, *Campylobacter*, *Yersinia,* and *Aeromonas*) and a test for *C difficile* should be done if any of the above stool studies is positive, or if a patient has any of the following:
  - Fever greater than 38.5° C
  - Severe diarrhea
  - Bloody stools
  - Persistent diarrhea that has not been treated empirically with an antimicrobial agent; noncholera *Vibrio* bacteria should also be sought in this setting.
- Stool testing for ova and parasites (O&P) should be ordered in the settings described in **Table 2.5**.

Special stool studies may be needed to identify certain organisms that will be missed by routine stool cultures, and testing should be done in the appropriate epidemiologic settings. These pathogens include enterohemorrhagic colitis-producing *E coli* 0157:H7, other shigatoxin-producing *E coli*, *Vibrio cholerae*, other noncholera *Vibrio* bacteria, some strains of *Yersinia,* and *C difficile*.

Endoscopy (flexible sigmoidoscopy or colonoscopy) should be done in patients with persistent diarrhea that has failed to respond to empiric therapy and in homosexual males with diarrhea.

■ **Supportive Treatment of Acute Diarrhea**

Fluid and electrolyte repletion is often the most important intervention in acute diarrhea. Adults in the greatest need of rehydration are the elderly and the immunosuppressed, as well as those with voluminous diarrhea.

TABLE 2.5 — HISTORICAL CLUES THAT STOOL TESTING FOR PARASITES IS INDICATED

Historical Clue	Parasite(s) Suspected
Persistent diarrhea	*Giardia*, *Cryptosporidium*, and amebae
Recent travel to mountainous areas or to recreational waters in the United States	*Giardia*
Recent trip to Russia	*Giardia*, *Cryptosporidium* or both
Recent trip to Nepal	*Cyclospora*
Exposure to infants in day-care centers	*Giardia* and *Cryptosporidium*
Homosexual male	*Giardia* and amebae
Patient with acquired immunodeficiency disease (AIDS)	*Cryptosporidium* parvum, *Isospora belli*, *Cyclospora*, and Microsporidia
Public waterborne outbreak	*Giardia* and *Cryptosporidium*
Bloody stools with few leukocytes	Amebae

Rehydration sources include:
- Pedialyte or other related solutions
- Sports drinks, diluted fruit juices, broths, and soups
- In cases of more severe diarrhea, oral rehydration solutions can be prepared as follows, and drunk alternately:
    - 8 oz orange, apple, or other fruit juice with ½ tsp honey or corn syrup and a pinch of salt
    - 8 oz water plus ¼ tsp of baking soda.

A recommended diet during acute diarrhea might include:
- Boiled and salted starches or cereals such as potatoes, noodles, rice, wheat, or oats
- Crackers, bananas, yogurt, soup, and boiled vegetables
- Dairy products may or may not be tolerated well.

■ Nonspecific Antidiarrheal Therapy

Drugs that slow the flow of liquid through the bowel thereby facilitating absorption are generally effective in controlling diarrhea once treatable infection has been excluded. Choices include:
- Loperamide (Imodium), 4 mg initially, then 2 mg after each loose stool to a maximum of 16 mg/day for no more than 2 days. This is the preferred drug due to its safety, lack of significant opiate side effects, and ability to reduce the number of bowel movements by about 80%.
- Diphenoxylate with atropine (Lomotil), 2 tablets qid for up to 2 days. This has much more of a central opiate effect and also may produce anticholinergic side effects from atropine.
- Tincture of opium, 0.5 to 1 mL po q 4 to 6 hours for up to 2 days, can be used when other anti-mo-

tility agents fail or if a liquid medication is needed. It may be useful in AIDS-related diarrhea.

- Bismuth subsalicylate (Pepto-Bismol) at doses of 30 mL or 2 tablets every 30 minutes for eight doses, then repeat the next day if needed. This is especially useful if vomiting predominates over diarrhea. It has an antisecretory effect on the colon and antidiarrheal properties that make it useful in prophylaxis against traveler's diarrhea.

- Attapulgite (Kaopectate) absorbs water as a claylike substance, making stools more formed. It is less effective than loperamide but is safe because it is not absorbed systemically.

- Octreotide acetate (Sandostatin) is a last-resort drug for refractory diarrhea because of the need to administer it parenterally (subcutaneously or intravenously) and its high cost. It has been utilized in the following conditions:
  – Pathogen-negative diarrhea
  – AIDS diarrhea
  – Ileostomy diarrhea
  – Diarrhea due to 5-fluorouracil chemotherapy
  – Microsporidia diarrhea.

■ **Selected Notes About Specific Therapy for Infectious Diarrhea**

Management considerations for various forms of infectious diarrhea (**Table 2.3**) include:

- *Shigella*: all confirmed cases should be treated with antibiotic therapy because the duration of the illness is shortened with treatment and because person-to-person spread occurs so readily (because of the small inoculum required to cause infection).

- *Salmonella*: healthy individuals with mild symptoms of intestinal infection should not receive antimicrobial therapy because it prolongs excretion of organisms. Bacteremia (occurring in up to 14% of cases) may result in systemic complications, and treatment should be reserved for those with risk factors (below), who have documented bacteremia, or who are ill enough to require hospitalization. Risk factors for bacteremia in salmonellosis include:

- Age: Infants <3 months or adults >65 years of age
- Human immunodeficiency virus (HIV) infection and AIDS
- Uremia
- Malignancies of all types
- After renal transplantation
- Other causes of immunodeficiency, including corticosteroid use

- Enterohemorrhagic *E coli* (EHEC) and *E coli* 0157:H7 should not be treated. Antibiotic therapy has been associated with an increased risk of the hemolytic uremic syndrome, attributed to toxin release from killed organisms.

■ Lactose Intolerance/Malabsorption

Lactose intolerance is a common cause of diarrhea and other postprandial symptoms, including flatulence and bloating. It is far more common in Asians and blacks (in whom up to 90% have some degree of jejunal lactase deficiency) than in whites (in whom only 5% to 15% are affected). This problem should be suspected when a patient associates symptoms with the intake of dairy products. Lactose malabsorption can easily be documented with a lactose-hydrogen breath test; the term *intolerance* is applied if symptoms are present. In young children, this diagnosis is virtually always secondary to another condition that damages the jejunal mucosa enough to result in lactase deficiency; however, in older patients, malabsorption is usually primary. The reason for the late onset of primary lactase deficiency in adults is unknown. An allergy to cow's milk protein must also be considered in patients with intolerance to dairy products.

The lactose-hydrogen breath test involves the ingestion of 50 g of a lactose solution, followed by serial measurement of breath hydrogen levels at half-hour intervals for 2 hours. An increase of at least 20 parts per million supports a diagnosis of malabsorption, although this does not distinguish small bowel bacterial overgrowth or other underlying causes from primary constitutional lactase deficiency.

Once lactose malabsorption is confirmed, management depends on the etiology. If a cause of secondary lactase deficiency can be identified, correction of the primary problem should be expected to resolve the lactose intolerance over a variable period of time. Milk allergy generally requires careful and thorough exclusion of all milk-containing products from the patient's diet. In the more commonly encountered situation of constitutional lactase deficiency, the patient should temporarily be restricted to a lactose-free diet (**Table 2.6**) for 2 to 4 weeks. This should clarify whether symptoms are due to lactose intolerance. If abstinence from lactose ingestion eliminates symptoms, the patient may benefit from commercial sources of β-D-galactosidase such as Lactaid, Lactrase, or Dairy Ease, which can be taken in tablet form before meals, or by adding these substances to milk at least 24 hours before use. Tablets provide between 3000 and 9000 U of lactase, and the number of tablets needed varies between individuals, depending on the extent of lactase deficiency. It may also be useful to have patients take one of these supplements before each meal during the trial of a lactose-free diet. Patients on a lactose-free diet should be reminded to take supplementation of at least 1000 to 1500 mg/day calcium to reduce the risk of osteoporosis.

TABLE 2.6 — FOODS TO BE AVOIDED IN A LACTOSE-FREE DIET*

- Any type of milk, including:
  - Whole
  - Skim
  - Evaporated
  - Condensed
  - Dried
  - Human breast
- Yogurt
- Milk-based drinks, such as:
  - Egg nog
  - Hot chocolate
- All cheeses
- Butter or margarine (unless specifically milk-free)
- Many commercial salad dressings
- Creamed soups or chowders
- Creamed or breaded meats, fish or poultry
- Many cold cuts, hot dogs, and other meat products that contain dried milk solids
- Many breads or baked products that contain dried milk solids, such as:
  - Muffins
  - Waffles
  - Doughnuts
- Candies, including:
  - Chocolate
  - Butterscotch
  - Toffee
- Some medications and nonprescription vitamins

* Food labels should be read carefully. Any foods containing any form of milk, dry milk solids, lactose, cream, or butter should be avoided.

■ *Clostridium difficile* Diarrhea

Responsible for many cases of antibiotic-associated diarrhea, its clinical presentation varies from a mild self-limited illness with diarrhea resolving soon after withdrawal of the offending antibiotic to a severe pseudomembranous colitis with fever, profuse watery (usually nonbloody) diarrhea and toxicity, with significant mortality. The small bowel is rarely affected by this organism. The diarrhea is often associated with fever, crampy abdominal pain, and leukocytosis. More serious complications include toxic megacolon and colonic perforation.

Risk Factors

Risk factors include:

- Antibiotic use within 4 to 8 weeks of presentation, especially:
  - Ampicillin
  - Amoxicillin
  - Clindamycin
  - Cephalosporins
- Hospitalization for any reason
- Recent surgery
- Uremia
- Crohn's disease
- Severe concurrent infection
- Recent cancer chemotherapy.

Diagnosis

Latex particle agglutination immunoassays are useful in detecting either the enterotoxin (toxin A) or the cytotoxin (toxin B) produced by *C difficile* in the stool, with up to 87% sensitivity and 99% to 100% specificity. This test is rapid (taking only 2 to 3 hours to process) and inexpensive.

The gold standard test is a tissue-culture assay for the cytotoxin, with sensitivity and specificity both near 100%, but utility of this test is limited by high cost and the requirement of overnight incubation.

Endoscopy can be done if the diagnosis remains in doubt. Sigmoidoscopy or colonoscopy will demonstrate pseudomembranes in half of documented cases (**Figures 2.1 and 2.2**).

FIGURE 2.1 — ENDOSCOPIC IMAGE OF PSEUDOMEMBRANOUS COLITIS

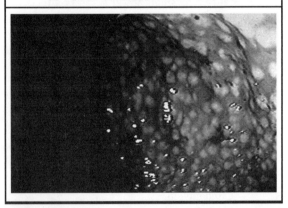

Management

The offending antibiotic should be discontinued, if possible. Milder symptoms are best left untreated, as they often resolve spontaneously. If the antibiotic must be continued or if symptoms are prolonged or severe, therapy can be given. Oral antibiotic therapy can be prescribed at the dosages shown for 10 to 14 days (**Table 2.7**). Patients who cannot take medication enterally can be treated with metronidazole 500 mg IV q 8 hours. Intravenous vancomycin is ineffective and should not be prescribed in this setting. Severe refractory colitis, toxic megacolon, or perforation may necessitate surgical resection (**Figure 2.3**).

Relapses are usually due to incomplete eradication of the initial infection rather than to antibiotic resistance. Mild relapses should not be treated, as this does not prevent subsequent relapses. More symptomatic relapses can be treated with metronidazole 500 mg po tid plus rifampin 300 mg po bid. Slow tapering of oral vancomycin is an alternative, but comparative trials of relapse treatment options have not been carried out.

FIGURE 2.2 — HISTOLOGIC PICTURE OF PSEUDOMEMBRANOUS COLITIS

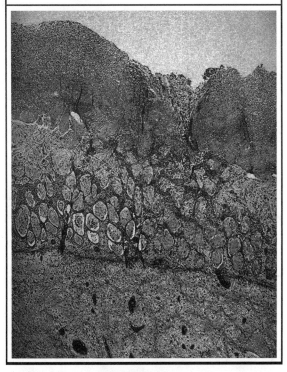

■ Diarrhea in the AIDS Patient

Diarrhea occurs in up to 90% of AIDS patients and can be responsible for dehydration, weight loss, malnutrition, and wasting. Its differential diagnosis is shown in **Table 2.2**, and the etiology can be predicted with some success based in part on the extent of immunosuppression. Persons with CD4$^+$ counts >400/mm^3 are more likely to have nonopportunistic infections with common organisms or noninfectious causes of diarrhea, eg, reaction to antiretroviral therapy, most notably the protease inhibitor nelfinavir. CD4$^+$ counts <100/mm^3 predispose one to opportunis-

TABLE 2.7 — INITIAL TREATMENT OPTIONS FOR *CLOSTRIDIUM DIFFICILE* DIARRHEA*

Drug	Response Rate (%)	Relapse Rate (%)
Metronidazole 500 mg po tid or 250 mg po qid	98	7
Vancomycin 125 mg po qid	96	18
Bacitracin 25,000 U po qid	83	34
Cholestyramine 4 g po tid	68	Unknown
* All given for 10 to 14 days.		

Adapted from: Kelly CP, et al. *N Engl J Med.* 1994;330: 257-262.

FIGURE 2.3 — SURGICAL SPECIMEN OF PSEUDOMEMBRANOUS COLITIS

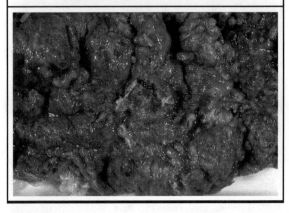

tic infections such as cytomegalovirus (CMV), *Mycobacterium avium* complex (MAC), fungi, and otherwise unusual protozoal infections. More than one pathogen is often responsible for symptoms, and their invasion is the best predictor of pathogenicity. Fulminant infections may occur, but usually only in the setting of extremely severe immunodeficiency (CD4$^+$ <50/mm^3). The evaluation in all cases should include stool studies, while endoscopic evaluation is restricted to specific indications (**Table 2.8**).

Acute infectious diarrhea is most commonly found to be due to Salmonella infection and, if antibiotics are being taken, *Clostridium difficile* infection. Chronic diarrhea, while often due to common organisms such as Campylobacter spp and *Giardia lamblia*, the most common opportunists involved are CMV,

---

**TABLE 2.8 — EVALUATION OF
DIARRHEA IN AIDS**

- Initial evaluation – stool collection for:
  - Culture for *Salmonella, Shigella,* and *Campylobacter*
  - WBCs
  - Sudan black B fat stain
  - *Clostridium difficile* testing
  - Ova and parasites (3 to 6 specimens)
  - Acid-fast bacterial staining *Cryptosporidium, Isospora,* and *Cyclospora*
  - Trichrome staining for Microsporidium
- If rectal bleeding, tenesmus or WBCs in stool specimen, sigmoidoscopy, or colonoscopy for:
  - Histologic biopsies (looking especially for viruses and protozoa)
  - Rectal biopsy for culture (for *Campylobacter* and possibly for viruses)
- If persistent unexplained diarrhea and weight loss, upper endoscopy for:
  - Duodenal aspirate (for bacteria and protozoa, including *Giardia*)
  - Bacterial culture of duodenal content
  - Small bowel biopsy (may diagnose MAC even if blood cultures are nondiagnostic)

Abbreviations: AIDS, acquired immunodeficiency syndrome; MAC, *Mycobacterium avium* complex; WBC, white blood cell.

Cryptosporidia, MAC, and Microsporidia (including *Enterocytozoon bieneusi* and *Encephalitozoon intestinalis)*. Diarrhea due to fungi (Histoplasmosis, cryptococcosis, and coccidioidomycosis) generally occurs in the context of systemic infection.

Highly active anti-retroviral therapy (HAART) directed toward the restoration of immune function often reduces the severity of infection, prevents relapses and often obviates the need for specific anti-infective therapy. With HAART, the need for maintenance anti-infective therapy (otherwise inevitably needed) can usually be avoided. HAART usually includes:

- A protease inhibitor
- A nucleoside analog (DNA chain terminator)
- Either a second nucleoside analog (often referred to as a "nuke") or a non-nucleoside reverse transcription inhibitor.

Management of specific infections in immuno-compromised patients (including those with AIDS) is summarized in **Table 2.9**. Symptomatic treatment of diarrhea may provide a significant improvement in quality of life, particularly when infection is not found or if infection responds poorly or slowly to specific therapy. Loperamide (Imodium), diphenoxylate with atropine (Lomotil), or deiodinated tincture of opium can be used. More refractory diarrhea may respond to subcutaneous octreotide (Sandostatin) at dosages of 50 to 500 µg tid.

Management of infectious diarrhea in immuno-compromised patients (including those with AIDS) is discussed in **Table 2.9**. Limited evaluation should be followed promptly by therapy (specific or nonspecific), reserving extensive evaluation for failures after treatment.

SUGGESTED READING

DuPont HL. Guidelines on acute infectious diarrhea in adults. The Practice Parameters Committee of the American College of Gastrogenterology. *Am J Gastroenterol.* 1997;92:1962-1975.

Gilbert DN, Moellering RC, Sande MA. *The Sanford Guide to Antimicrobial Therapy 2003.* 33rd ed. Hyde Park, Vt: Antimicrobial Therapy, Inc; 2003.

Kelly CP, Pothoulakis C, LaMont JT. *Clostridium difficile* colitis. *N Engl J Med.* 1994;330:257-262.

Wilcox CM. Gastrointestinal manifestations of the acquired immunodeficiency syndrome. In: Feldman M, Friedman LS, Sleisenger MH, eds. *Sleisenger and Fordtran's Gastrointestinal and Liver Disease*: *Pathophysiology/Diagnosis/Management.* 7th ed. Philadelphia, Pa: WB Saunders Co; 2002.

TABLE 2.9 — TREATMENT OF INFECTIOUS DIARRHEA IN IMMUNOCOMPROMISED PATIENTS

Indication for Antibiotic Treatment	Suggested Antibiotic Treatment*
Shigellosis	Ciprofloxacin 500 mg po bid or ofloxacin 300 mg po bid for 7-10 days
Salmonellosis (nontyphi)	Ciprofloxacin 500 mg po bid for 5-7 days, or azithromycin 1 g po once then 500 mg po daily for 6 days
Clostridium difficile colitis	See Table 2.7; treat for 10-14 days
Cryptosporidium diarrhea	HAART alone; if ineffective, use nitazoxanide (Cryptaz) 0.5-1.0 g po bid (or combination of paromomycin 1 g po bid + azithromycin 600 mg po daily) + antidiarrheal therapy.
Isospora diarrhea	TMP/SMX 160/800 mg po qid for 10 days, then bid for 3 weeks
Cyclospora cayatanensis diarrhea	TMP/SMX 160/800 mg po qid for 10 d, then same dose once 3 times a week indefinitely

Microsporidiosis	Albendazole 400 mg po bid for 3 weeks (effective for *E intestinalis* but not for *E bieneusi*); oral fumagillin 60 mg po daily for 2 weeks was effective for *E bieneusi* in a small study
Mycobacterium avium complex	HAART + multidrug regimen including clarithromycin 500 mg po bid (or azithromycin 600 mg po daily) + ethambutol 15-25 mg/kg po daily + one or more of the following: ciprofloxacin 750 mg po bid, rifabutin 300 mg po daily, ofloxacin 400 mg po bid, and amikacin 7.5 – 15 mg/kg IV daily; this must be followed with suppressive therapy indefinitely (unless HAART results in adequate restoration of CD4 count) with ethambutol 15 mg/kg po daily and either clarithromycin 500 mg po bid or azithromycin 600 mg po daily
Small bowel bacterial overgrowth	Ciprofloxacin 500 mg po bid (or TMP/SMX 160/800 mg po bid) for 3-5 days
Cytomegalovirus	Induction therapy for 3-6 weeks with valganciclovir 900 mg po bid with food or ganciclovir 5 mg/kg IV q 12 hours or foscarnet 90 mg/kg IV q12 hours, then maintenance (suppressive) therapy with valganciclovir 900 mg po daily or ganciclovir 5 mg/kg IV daily or 6 mg/kg IV daily 5 days per week or foscarnet 90-120 mg/kg IV daily
Herpes simplex virus	Acyclovir 5 mg/kg IV q 8 hours for 7 days or 400 mg po 5 times a day for 14-21 days or famciclovir 500 mg po bid for 7 days

Continued

Indication for Antibiotic Treatment	Suggested Antibiotic Treatment*
Histoplasmosis	For less severe disease: Itraconazole 300 mg po bid for 3 days, then 200 mg po bid for 12 weeks or 400 mg po daily for 12 weeks, then 200 mg daily. *For moderate to severe disease:* Liposomal amphotericin B 3 mg/kg/d IV for 14 days, then itraconazole 200 mg po daily or amphotericin B 0.5-1 mg/kg/d IV for 7 days, then 0.8 mg/kg/d IV qod to total dose of 10-15 mg/kg then itraconazole 200 mg po daily
Cryptococcosis	Treatment with either IV amphotericin B or po fluconazole is given in the context of systemic infection
Coccidioidomycosis	Treatment with either IV amphotericin B or po itraconazole is given in the context of systemic infection

Abbreviations: HAART, highly active antiretroviral therapy; IV, intravenous; TMP/SMX, trimethoprim/sulfamethoxazole.

* This table lists regimens used commonly in early 2003; in many situations alternative regimens are available. Doses of medications assume normal renal function. Information adapted from: *The Sanford Guide to Antimicrobial Therapy 2003.*

3

Diarrhea: Chronic

Chronic or recurrent diarrhea, defined as lasting more than 4 weeks, is most commonly due to:
- Irritable bowel syndrome
- Inflammatory bowel disease
- Malabsorption
- Parasitic infection.

Surreptitious laxative abuse or factitious diarrhea should also be considered. Many causes of acute diarrhea may also persist chronically, thus the evaluation should first exclude these diagnoses. The causes of most cases of chronic diarrhea are listed in **Table 3.1**.

Irritable bowel syndrome (functional diarrhea) should be distinguished from organic disease before embarking on a complicated evaluation of chronic diarrhea. Organic disease can be predicted with 90% certainty if at least three of the following clinical and laboratory parameters are present:
- Sudden definable onset of symptoms with daily occurrence
- Nocturnal symptoms
- Duration <3 months
- Weight loss of >12 lbs (5 kg)
- Average daily stool volume >400 g.

Chronic diarrhea can be subdivided based on whether the mechanism of diarrhea is osmotic or secretory, although many cases will have evidence of both mechanisms. A 24- to 48-hour fast should temporarily eliminate osmotic diarrhea, while secretory diarrhea should continue unabated. If fasting is impossible or

TABLE 3.1 — MAJOR CAUSES OF CHRONIC DIARRHEA

No Previous Evaluation
- Irritable bowel syndrome
- Inflammatory bowel disease
- Ischemic bowel disease
- Chronic bacterial/mycobacterial infections
- Parasitic and fungal infections
- Bacterial overgrowth
- Radiation enteritis
- Malabsorption syndromes
- Medications
- Alcohol
- Intestinal lymphoma
- Pancreatic insufficiency
- Colon cancer
- Villous adenoma
- Previous surgery:
  - Gastrectomy
  - Vagotomy
  - Intestinal resection
  - Cholecystectomy
- Endocrine causes:
  - Hyperthyroidism
  - Hypothyroidism
  - Hypoparathyroidism
  - Addison's disease (adrenal insufficiency)
  - Diabetes mellitus
  - Pheochromocytoma
  - Ganglioneuroma
- Fecal impaction
- Heavy metal poisoning
- "Brainerd diarrhea" — chronic epidemic diarrhea due to the digestion of unpasteurized milk

impractical, a measurement of the stool osmotic gap can be done.

The stool osmotic gap = $290 - 2([Na+] + [K+])$ where $[Na+] + [K+]$ are the stool concentrations of sodium and potassium, respectively, based on a normal osmolality of blood and stool of 290 mOsm/kg. An osmolar gap of <50 is typical of a pure secretory diarrhea, while a pure osmotic diarrhea is associated with an elevated gap, usually >125. Carbohydrate malabsorption or a mixed osmotic and secretory diarrhea will result in an osmotic gap between 50 and 125. For the measured osmolality to be accurate, the stool specimen should be evaluated promptly or refrigerated. Bacterial activity in a recently collected and unrefrigerated specimen will falsely increase the stool osmolality, and a stool osmolality measured at much <290 mOsm/kg indicates that the stool has been diluted, either inadvertently by urine or by intentionally diluting it with water or urine to create factitious diarrhea. If the accuracy of stool osmolality is in question, the serum osmolality should be checked and compared with the measured stool value.

Initial Evaluation of Chronic Diarrhea

A stool specimen should be obtained for:
- Direct visual examination (for oil, blood, and mucus)
- White blood cells
- Occult blood
- Sudan black B fat stain
- Ova and parasites
- Electrolytes and osmolality (to determine osmotic gap)
- pH (<5.3 suggests carbohydrate malabsorption)
- Alkalization (for phenolphthalein-containing laxatives).

Blood studies should be obtained for:
- Complete blood count
- Erythrocyte sedimentation rate
- Thyroid function studies.

Colonoscopy or flexible sigmoidoscopy with biopsies may be performed for direct mucosal examination, which may demonstrate melanosis coli (usually due to the use of anthracene-containing laxatives), inflammation (colitis), ulceration and polyps, or masses. Biopsies may enable one to diagnose collagenous colitis, lymphocytic colitis, amyloidosis, Crohn's disease, ulcerative colitis, cancer, and some infections.

Less often, there may be the need for an upper gastrointestinal endoscopy for small bowel biopsy and possibly for a duodenal aspirate, checking for:
- *Giardia*
- Crohn's disease
- Celiac disease
- Intestinal lymphoma
- Eosinophilic gastroenteritis
- Whipple's disease
- Various infections.

A small-bowel series or small-bowel enema (enteroclysis) is sometimes helpful in evaluating for Crohn's disease, jejunal diverticula (which predispose to bacterial overgrowth), and fistulas. Computed tomography (CT) or ultrasound examination of the abdomen and pelvis may be performed. A 72-hour stool collection for weight and for quantitative fat content may aid in the evaluation. Daily stool fat should be <7 g in a patient on a diet containing 100 g of fat per day.

A therapeutic trial of a lactose-free diet may be helpful (see Chapter 2, *Diarrhea: Acute Diarrhea and Diarrhea in AIDS*, Lactose Intolerance/Malabsorption section). An empiric trial of metronidazole (for bacterial overgrowth and for giardiasis) or ciprofloxacin may be therapeutic prior to embarking on a detailed evaluation for rare causes of chronic diarrhea. Bacterial overgrowth due to stasis from jejunal diverticula, surgical bypass procedures, or dysmotility may respond well to appropriate antibiotic therapy.

Selected Chronic Diarrheal States

■ Dumping Syndrome

The dumping syndrome after gastrectomy and/or vagotomy is mainly associated with truncal (rather than selective) vagotomy. Rapid emptying of hyperosmolar gastric content into the small bowel obligates large amounts of fluid to be secreted into the intestinal lumen, combined with release of enteric neuropeptides. Symptoms of early dumping (within 30 minutes of a meal) include:

- Diarrhea
- Orthostatic dizziness
- Flushing
- Nausea
- Abdominal pain.

Late dumping (several hours after a meal) is attributed to hypoglycemia and the rapid emptying of carbohydrate into the small intestine accompanied by physiologic hyperinsulinemia. The carbohydrate is cleared from the intestine before the elevated insulin level normalizes, resulting in hypoglycemia. Symptoms include:

- Anxiety
- Tremulousness
- Palpitations
- Confusion
- Diaphoresis.

Management includes reduced intake of simple sugars, ingestion of liquids and solids separately, and a diet divided into frequent small meals. Octreotide, a somatostatin analogue, may help in patients who do not respond to the postvagotomy diet by inhibiting insulin and neuropeptide secretion.

■ Ileostomy Diarrhea

Ileostomy diarrhea may occur after total colectomy and terminal ileal resection. The typical stool output through an end ileostomy is about 500 g (about twice the maximum output without surgery). A larger output results from longer segments of ileum being resected, due to malabsorption of water, electrolytes, vitamin B_{12}, various nutrients, and bile salts. This may be due to partial small bowel obstruction, recurrent Crohn's disease, or bacterial overgrowth in the proximal portion of the small intestine.

Treatment may be nonspecific:

- Loperamide, diphenoxylate-atropine, or codeine
- Increasing fluid, salt, and sugar intake
- Treating bacterial overgrowth with trimethoprim/sulfamethoxazole (TMP/SMX), metronidazole, a tetracycline, or a fluoroquinolone
- Parenteral octreotide.

Pouchitis involves inflammation of the ileostomy site in ulcerative colitis patients and may be associated with extraintestinal symptoms. It is likely due either to anaerobic bacterial overgrowth or to recurrent inflammatory bowel disease in the pouch. If metronidazole does not resolve symptoms, sulfasalazine, 5-aminosalicylates, or corticosteroids may be effective. Dietary fat reduction is needed if there is significant steatorrhea. Octreotide may be useful in reducing output, but surgery may be needed if obstruction or peritonitis ensue.

■ Diabetic Diarrhea

Up to 20% of long-standing insulin-dependent diabetics will complain of chronic diarrhea. Passage of frequent watery stools may occur, especially at night or when supine. Steatorrhea, usually mild but occasionally severe, may occur without cachexia or significant weight loss. Other signs of autonomic neuropathy are often present, and this is thought to cause bowel dysmotility as an explanation for the diarrhea.

Treatment options include:
- Clonidine (tablets or transdermal patch)
- Oxybutynin (also used to control bladder spasms)
- Cholestyramine
- Antibiotics (if bacterial overgrowth is responsible for the diarrhea)
- Opiates such as codeine.

Tighter glycemic control may reduce this complication of diabetes.

■ Microscopic Colitis (Collagenous Colitis and Lymphocytic Colitis)

These colitides cause chronic watery diarrhea and are most often diagnosed in middle-aged women. Biopsies of an endoscopically normal-appearing colon will reveal inflammatory changes under a microscope. A thickened subepithelial collagen band (7 to 100 µm rather than 1 to 7 µm as in normals) (**Figure 3.1**) is the hallmark of collagenous colitis, along with epithelial lymphocyte infiltration. When the thickened collagen band is absent, the term "microscopic colitis" or, more recently, "lymphocytic colitis" is used.

FIGURE 3.1 — COLLAGENOUS COLITIS

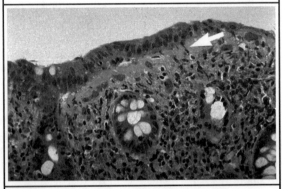

Thickened subepithelial collagen layer (arrow).

Pathogenesis involves intraepithelial T lymphocytes which may be interacting with an unidentified luminal antigen, although this has not been confirmed.

Treatment is usually initiated with simple antidiarrheal medication, with progression to other therapy if the initial choice is ineffective. Aminosalicylates (balsalazide, mesalamine, or sulfasalazine) then cholestyramine should be utilized before considering the use of corticosteroids. Other immunosuppressive agents such as methotrexate, 6-mercaptopurine, or azathioprine have rarely been needed to avoid colectomy.

■ Factitious Diarrhea

Diarrhea may be self-induced with laxatives, or patients may simulate diarrhea by adding water, urine, or other liquid to their stools. This is often seen in association with eating disorders, such as anorexia nervosa and bulimia nervosa, in an effort to control body weight. Other patients with factitious diarrhea will simulate diarrhea to expose themselves to extensive medical evaluation, possibly for secondary gain.

This diagnosis requires suspicion on the part of the health-care provider, and can be approached clinically by checking the stool for phenolphthalein (by alkalinizing a stool specimen), finding melanosis coli or hyperpigmentation of the colonic wall due to anthracene laxative such as senna or cascara, or finding a fecal osmolality to be much <290 mOsm/kg. The ultimate confirmatory finding, of course, is a room search, in which laxatives are found in a patient's home or hospital room.

■ Diarrhea in the Intensive Care Unit

The most common causes of diarrhea in patients in the intensive care unit (ICU) include:

- Antibiotic therapy (side effect from loss of colonic flora needed to ferment carbohydrates) or *Clostridium difficile* colitis
- Other infections
- Sorbitol in elixir medications (eg, theophylline)
- Magnesium-containing antacids
- H_2 receptor antagonists
- Cancer chemotherapy agents
- Fecal impaction
- Intestinal ischemia
- Intolerance of enteral nutritional supplements (infrequent).

Enteral supplements may be poorly tolerated because of high osmolality of some formulas, rapid infusion, rapid transit due to motility irregularity, partial villous atrophy due to prolonged periods of taking nothing by mouth, preexisting malabsorption, bacterial contamination of the tube feeding formula, or stimulation of proximal colonic secretion of water. Slowing the rate of infusion of enteral nutrition may be helpful, though dilution of the formula usually is ineffective. A high-fiber formula (Jevity) is of unpredictable benefit.

■ Chronic Diarrhea of Unknown Origin

An exhaustive diagnostic evaluation may fail to reach a diagnosis to explain chronic diarrhea in some cases. In this scenario, the most common diagnoses are:
- Surreptitious laxative abuse
- Drug- or food-induced diarrhea
- Incontinence due to anal sphincter dysfunction
- Irritable bowel syndrome
- Collagenous or lymphocytic (microscopic) colitis
- Unrecognized malabsorption
- Idiopathic bile acid malabsorption.

Small bowel malabsorption or pancreatic insufficiency may occasionally be found to be the cause of chronic diarrhea and should be considered particularly if there is unexplained fat in a stool specimen. The D-xylose test can be used as an indicator of proximal small-bowel malabsorption of carbohydrates. D-xylose is ingested and subsequently blood is drawn and a 5-hour urine collection is taken. Reduced serum or urinary content of xylose supports the possibility of reduced intestinal absorption. Hydrogen breath testing for xylose or lactose malabsorption may then be indicated for further evaluation.

The Schilling test evaluates the absorption of radiolabeled oral vitamin B_{12}, which may be impaired for a variety of reasons, including pernicious anemia (with failure of the stomach to produce intrinsic factor), pancreatic exocrine insufficiency, small-bowel bacterial overgrowth, or terminal ileal disease. In the absence of a gastrectomy or ileal resection, results of the Schilling test often help to determine the level at which malabsorption may be occurring. Results of the Schilling test after a course of an antibiotic, a trial of pancreatic enzymes, or the administration of oral intrinsic factor (the second stage of the Schilling test) can more effectively explain the reason for malabsorption.

Pancreatic function can be assessed by a variety of studies when the reason for malabsorptive diarrhea remains obscure. These include:

- The secretin test: testing the response of the pancreas to a stimulus such as intravenous secretin (requires nasoenteric intubation)
- Measurement of fecal chymotrypsin concentration (where available)
- The bentiromide test in which a synthetic chemical is ingested and the urine is collected to measure the excretion of its metabolite, para-aminobenzoic acid (PABA); normal pancreatic function is required to produce PABA.

If no diagnosis can be made, the term "idiopathic chronic diarrhea" is used. This condition typically regresses and clears in a matter of months to years.

4 IBS: General Information

The irritable bowel syndrome (IBS) is a combination of chronic or recurrent gastrointestinal (GI) symptoms not explained by structural or biochemical abnormalities. The usual symptoms are attributed to dysmotility of the intestinal tract and include:

- Abdominal pain
- Disturbed defecation
  - Constipation
  - Diarrhea
  - Alternating periods of constipation and diarrhea
- Bloating
- Distention.

Irritable bowel syndrome is a diagnosis of exclusion made on a clinical basis, lacking a specific confirmatory diagnostic test. By definition, tests of intestinal structure (such as sigmoidoscopy and colonic biopsies) are normal, and IBS is considered to be a "functional bowel disease." Although IBS does not predispose one to potentially more serious organic diseases such as colitis or colon cancer, individuals affected by IBS have an impaired quality of life, significant impairment in functional status, more frequent disability claims, and greater work absenteeism; they also require more doctor visits than the general population.

In Great Britain and the United States, IBS affects 14% to 24% of women and 5% to 19% of men. There is usually a lower reporting frequency of IBS in older age groups. A similar frequency exists among blacks and whites, while it is less common in the Hispanic population.

In more than half of patients, the first presentation of symptoms occurs between 30 and 50 years of age. IBS is the second most frequently encountered diagnosis in clinical practice, accounting for more physician visits than any symptoms except for those of respiratory tract infections, and it is the most frequent diagnosis made in a typical gastroenterologist's practice. It accounts for 12% of primary care visits and 28% of gastroenterology visits. Although IBS accounts for 2.4 to 3.5 million visits annually to physicians and for 2.2 million prescriptions in the United States, up to 70% of people with IBS symptoms do not seek medical attention.

Pathophysiology

Irritable bowel syndrome causes a dysregulation in the functions of the intestinal motor, sensory and central nervous systems. Symptoms of IBS usually are a response to:

- Disruption of the GI tract from infection
- Dietary indiscretions (eg, increased fat or alcohol intake)
- Lifestyle changes (eg, traveling or vigorous physical activity)
- Psychological stress.

Symptoms caused by IBS are due both to disturbances in intestinal motility and enhanced visceral sensitivity. Baseline small-bowel and colonic motility patterns in IBS are similar to those in healthy controls. Some patients with diarrhea-predominant IBS have accelerated transit in the small bowel and/or colon, while some with constipation-predominant IBS have slowed or delayed transit. There is increased motility in response to environmental or enteric stimuli, such as:

- Stress
- Meals
- Balloon dilatation
- Cholecystokinin.

Many IBS patients have enhanced visceral sensitivity (hyperalgesia). They are aware of distention and experience painful symptoms at pressures and volumes that are significantly lower than in control subjects. This distinction persists even after controlling for neuroticism. Despite these symptoms, IBS patients typically have a normal or even increased threshold for painful stimulation of somatic neuroreceptors. Patients with IBS often have an:

- Increased awareness of normal physiologic functions (including normal phasic bowel contractions)
- Increased sensitivity to painful distention in the small bowel and colon
- Atypical area of somatic referral of visceral pain.

Some patients with constipation-predominant IBS appear to have vagal dysfunction, while some with diarrhea-predominant IBS have sympathetic adrenergic dysfunction.

A history of physical or sexual abuse, major loss (eg, death or divorce), or other major trauma precedes the onset of IBS symptoms in a significant number of patients. People with IBS symptoms who do not seek medical attention tend to be psychologically similar to normal controls, while those who frequently see physicians often have psychological disturbances. A psychological stressor may produce symptoms through changes in intestinal physiologic function or indirectly as a purely psychological event (**Figure 4.1**).

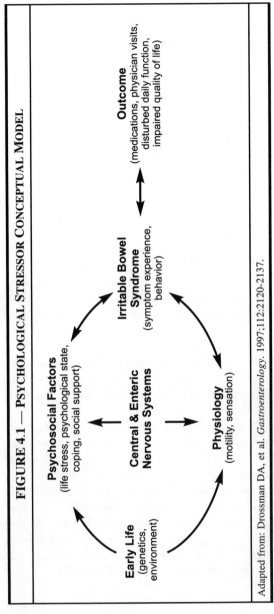

FIGURE 4.1 — PSYCHOLOGICAL STRESSOR CONCEPTUAL MODEL

Psychosocial Factors
(life stress, psychological state, coping, social support)

Central & Enteric Nervous Systems

Physiology
(motility, sensation)

Irritable Bowel Syndrome
(symptom experience, behavior)

Outcome
(medications, physician visits, disturbed daily function, impaired quality of life)

Early Life
(genetics, environment)

Adapted from: Drossman DA, et al. *Gastroenterology.* 1997;112:2120-2137.

SUGGESTED READING

American Gastroenterological Association. American Gastroenterological Association medical position statement: irritable bowel syndrome. *Gastroenterology*. 1997;112:2118-2119.

Delvaux M. Role of visceral sensitivity in the pathophysiology of irritable bowel syndrome. *Gut*. 2002;51(suppl 1):I67-I71.

Drossman DA, Whitehead WE, Camilleri M. Irritable bowel syndrome: a technical review for practice guideline development. *Gastroenterology*. 1997;112:2120-2137.

4

5   IBS: Diagnosis

A sequential diagnostic strategy for the irritable bowel syndrome (IBS) includes:

- Symptom-based diagnostic criteria
- Conservative evaluation strategy based on predominant symptoms
- Initiation of symptomatic treatment with prompt reassessment.

Symptom-Based Diagnostic Criteria

A unified set of criteria (the Rome Criteria) is utilized for symptom assessment (**Table 5.1**) as are the older Manning Criteria (**Table 5.2**).

Abdominal pain is the most common symptom of IBS. Pain is most commonly located in the left lower quadrant of the abdomen. It may be incited by eating anything (via an exaggerated "gastrocolic reflex"), and at least temporarily may be relieved by defecation. It is often exacerbated by colonic distention and stressful situations. Pain generally does not awaken the patient from sleep.

Abdominal distention (bloating) and related symptoms of belching and flatus are more often due to heightened sensitivity to distention than to an abnormally large amount of gas produced in the bowel. Distention and bloating are often relieved with passage of flatus or with belching.

Altered bowel habits are frequently reported, such as alternating constipation and diarrhea or the predominance of one of these symptoms. Some patients may have extended periods of constipation, interspersed

TABLE 5.1 — ROME CRITERIA FOR SYMPTOM ASSESSMENT OF IRRITABLE BOWEL SYNDROME

- At least 3 months of continuous or recurrent symptoms* of the following:
  - Abdominal pain or discomfort:
    - Relieved with defecation, or
    - Associated with a change in stool frequency, or
    - Associated with a change in stool consistency
- Two or more of the following, at least on 25% of occasions or days:
  - Altered stool frequency (for research purposes, "altered" may be defined as more than three bowel movements each day or less then three bowel movements each week), or
  - Altered stool form (lumpy/hard or loose/watery stool), or
  - Altered stool passage (straining, urgency, or feeling of incomplete evaluation), or
  - Passage of mucus, or
  - Bloating or feeling of abdominal distention

* Evaluation also includes a complete physical examination, sigmoidoscopy, and additional testing when indicated. Other recommended studies include examination of the stool (for ova and parasites, occult blood, laxatives), complete blood count, erythrocyte sedimentation rate, and serum chemistries. In certain cases, imaging studies (eg, upper gastrointestinal series, colonoscopy with rectal biopsy) will be needed.

with brief occasions of diarrhea, or constipation and diarrhea may alternate on a more frequent basis.

Diarrhea often occurs as small volumes of loose stool at frequent intervals. Urgency or tenesmus often precede bowel movements and may or may not be relieved by defecation. Diarrhea may be associated with the passage of flatus. The patient will often have no more than three stools per day (the upper limit of nor-

> ## TABLE 5.2 — MANNING CRITERIA FOR SYMPTOM ASSESSMENT OF IRRITABLE BOWEL SYNDROME
>
> - Abdominal pain relieved by defecation
> - Looser stools with onset of pain
> - More frequent stools with onset of pain
> - Abdominal distention
> - Passage of mucus in stools
> - Sensation of incomplete evacuation

mal frequency), but frequency may increase from baseline during flares of symptoms.

Constipation is objectively defined as fewer than three bowel movements weekly and is subjectively described as difficult or painful evacuation. Constipation often begins in childhood or many years before IBS is diagnosed. Stools may be hard and pellet-like (scybalous) due to exaggerated colonic haustral contractions or narrow in caliber (pencil-like) due to colonic and rectal spasm. Constipation may result in chronic laxative abuse.

Patients with IBS may note increased stool mucus; it may be clear or whitish. The etiology of this mucus is not understood, but it is not due to local inflammation.

Upper gastrointestinal (GI) symptoms may be seen in up to 50% of patients diagnosed with IBS and include:

- Pyrosis
- Dyspepsia
- Nausea
- Vomiting.

Exacerbation of IBS symptoms may occur during menstruation. They are often most prominent at the beginning of the menstrual cycle when there are elevated serum levels of prostaglandins E_2 and F_2; thus prostaglandins may be mediators.

Stress and tension often precede and trigger symptoms of IBS. The relationship of stress to GI symptoms may date back to childhood. Many IBS patients have an associated major clinical psychiatric disorder that either precedes or coincides with the diagnosis of IBS, if evaluated. Depression, anxiety, and, especially, panic disorders are frequently associated with IBS. Treatment of the psychiatric disorder is effective, providing the patient with emotional relief; more than half of patients will experience an improvement in GI symptoms.

Irritable bowel syndrome patients are often more preoccupied with illness than are controls. They tend to report more unrelated illnesses and tend to be more debilitated from other illnesses than controls.

Other clinical factors to be considered when diagnosing IBS include:

- Duration and severity of symptoms; more severe or more disabling symptoms or those that are more recent in onset are reasons for more extensive evaluation
- Change over time
- Demographics: IBS is more common in women and in younger patients
- Referral status of patient: patients seen in primary care settings are less likely to require extensive evaluation than are those whose condition is more severe who are referred to subspecialists
- Previous diagnostic evaluations
- A family history of colon cancer, especially if it occurred at a younger age
- Nature and extent of psychosocial difficulties.

Clinical Features

Symptoms supporting the diagnosis of IBS in patients include:

- Lower abdominal pain:
  - Aggravated by meals
  - Relieved by defecation
  - More frequent bowel movements with onset of pain
  - Looser stools with onset of pain
  - Pain that does not awaken patient from sleep
- Visible abdominal distention
- Small stools (with constipation or diarrhea)
- Chronic symptoms consistent in pattern but variable in severity
- Symptoms that worsen during periods of stress.

In assessing the differential diagnosis of IBS, the following symptoms provide an argument against IBS:

- Onset of symptoms in older age
- Steady progressive course
- Frequent awakening by symptoms
- Fever
- Weight loss
- Rectal bleeding from other than fissures or internal hemorrhoids
- Anemia
- Steatorrhea (excessive amounts of fat in stools).

Physical Examination

Physical examination of a patient with suspected IBS is used mainly to exclude other organic diagnoses; the physician will usually find the examination of a patient with IBS to be normal. The patient may be observed to be tense or anxious. A tender sigmoid colon or tenderness to rectal examination may help in establishing the diagnosis of IBS. A basic profile of diagnostic studies directed toward confirming or excluding organic disease should be performed. It should include, but not be limited to:

- A white blood cell (WBC) count
- An erythrocyte sedimentation rate (ESR)
- Endoscopic and possibly radiographic evaluation of the large bowel (**Figure 5.1**).

If anal dysmotility is suspected based on examination, anorectal and pelvic floor tests (motility testing and defecography, respectively) may be indicated.

Additional initial testing is based on the predominant symptom:

- If diarrhea:
  - Lactose H_2 breath testing
  - Testing of stools for WBCs and infection

FIGURE 5.1 — BASIC DIAGNOSIS OF IRRITABLE BOWEL SYNDROME

Symptom Assessment
(Rome Criteria)
(see Table 5.1)

Limited Screen for Organic Disease

- Hematology (complete blood count with WBC differential)
- Erythrocyte sedimentation rate (ESR)
- Thyroid function studies
- Stool testing for occult blood
- Stool examined for ova and parasites
- Flexible sigmoidoscopy ± barium enema or colonoscopy if >50 years of age or if inflammatory bowel disease is suspected in a younger patient

- Small-bowel series
- Consider a 24- to 48-hour fast to distinguish osmotic diarrhea (which should remit) from secretory diarrhea (which persists)
- If pain/gas/bloating: plain abdominal x-rays
- If painful defecation or fecal incontinence: anorectal motility testing
- If suggestion of bowel obstruction: plain x-rays or a barium small-bowel series
- If prominent upper-GI symptoms: upper-GI endoscopy and, if negative, consider ultrasound examination of the gall bladder.

Finding the following laboratory features would rule against IBS in the differential diagnosis process:
- Elevated ESR
- Leukocytosis
- Blood, pus, or fat in stool
- Stool weight greater than 200 g/day
- Persistent diarrhea during 48-hour fast (indicates a secretory diarrhea)
- Hypokalemia
- Motility testing failing to show spastic response to rectal distention.

Alternative diagnoses to be considered when diarrhea is present with a normal preliminary evaluation include:
- Osmotic diarrhea (due to ingestion of substances that are poorly digested):
  - Lactose intolerance is very common and should be excluded:
    - 2-Week lactose-free diet can be recommended (see Chapter 2, *Diarrhea: Acute Diarrhea and Diarrhea in AIDs*, Lactose Intolerance/Malabsorption section)
    - Alternatively can give trial of lactase supplement (eg, Lactaid milk)

- Specific testing can be done by hydrogen breath testing or a lactose tolerance test
  – Laxative abuse (eg, lactulose or mannitol)
  – Inadvertent excessive ingestion of laxatives (ie, sorbitol in sugar-free candy)
- Secretory diarrhea (persistence of diarrhea despite prolonged fasting):
  – May be caused by stimulatory laxatives such as Ex-Lax or Correctol
  – May require a home or hospital room search to clearly identify a laxative abuser
  – Human immunodeficiency virus (HIV) may be present without other symptoms
  – Pancreatic insufficiency or short-bowel syndrome (after extensive small-bowel surgery or radiation) should be considered in appropriate settings
- Inflammatory causes of diarrhea:
  – Ulcerative colitis: typically causes bleeding and can be readily diagnosed with sigmoidoscopy (see Chapter 10, *Ulcerative Colitis*)
  – Crohn's disease: may include systemic symptoms (fever, weight loss) but may be difficult to differentiate from IBS (see Chapter 11, *Crohn's Disease*)
  – Parasitic infections (especially giardiasis or amebiasis); unusual in absence of history of exposure:
    - Stool testing (3 separate specimens) should be done initially
    - Diagnosis of giardiasis may require a duodenal aspirate (by endoscopy or by a "string test")
- Endocrinopathies:
  – Addison's disease (adrenal insufficiency) may cause diarrhea in crisis
  – Hyperthyroidism may cause frequent formed stools (more often than watery stools).

The differential diagnosis of constipation with normal initial evaluation may include:

- Side effect of many medications:
  - Adrenergic agents
  - Anticholinergic drugs
  - Antihypertensive drugs
  - Narcotics
  - Antidepressant drugs
- Tolerance to effect of laxatives after chronic abuse
- Endocrinopathies:
  - Hypothyroidism
  - Hypoparathyroidism
- Colon cancer (especially in older patients or if symptoms are of recent onset)
- Diverticulitis or painful diverticulosis
- Factitious constipation, due to use of anti-diarrheals, narcotics, or anticholinergics.

SUGGESTED READING

Longstreth GF. Irritable bowel syndrome. Diagnosis in the managed care era. *Dig Dis Sci*. 1997;42:1105-1111.

Read NW. Irritable bowel syndrome. In: Feldman M, Friedman LS, Sleisenger MH, eds. *Sleisenger and Fordtran's Gastrointestinal and Liver Disease*: *Pathophysiology/Diagnosis/Management*. 7th ed. Philadelphia, Pa: WB Saunders Co; 2002:1794-1806.

6

IBS: Management

An initial treatment of irritable bowel syndrome (IBS) is outlined in **Table 6.1**. When this treatment fails, a protocol for further treatment is listed in **Table 6.2**.

A therapeutic relationship between the physician and patient may partially explain the high placebo response rate of 30% to 88%. The physician must determine a patient's understanding of the illness and his/her concerns. A thorough explanation of the disorder should be provided to the patient, clarifying that while IBS has a serious effect on one's quality of life, it does not lead to more serious conditions such as colitis or cancer.

The physician should respond to the patient's concerns and expectations by setting realistic and consistent limits. Involve the patient in the treatment plan. Establish a long-term relationship with the patient with more frequent visits initially, then at decreasing intervals. Reinforce the need for a relationship between the patient and the clinician. Determine the immediate reasons for a patient's visit:

- New exacerbating factors (dietary change, concurrent medical disorder, or side effect of new medication)
- Personal concern about a serious disease
- Environmental stressors, such as major loss or abuse history
- Psychiatric comorbidity (eg, depression, anxiety, or panic)
- Impairment in daily function
- Hidden agenda, such as narcotic or laxative abuse, pending disability, or secondary gain.

TABLE 6.1 — INITIAL TREATMENT OF IRRITABLE BOWEL SYNDROME*

Symptomatic Subgroup	Constipation	Diarrhea	Pain/Gas/Bloating
Review diet history	Yes	Yes	Yes
Additional tests	No	Lactose H_2 breath test	Plain abdominal x-ray
Therapeutic trial	Increase fiber; osmotic laxative	Loperamide (Imodium)	Antispasmodic

*Initiate treatment and reassess in 3 to 6 wk.

TABLE 6.2 — WHEN INITIAL TREATMENT OF IRRITABLE BOWEL SYNDROME FAILS

- Constipation:
  - Colonic transit test
  - Anal manometry and balloon expulsion
  - Measure anorectal angle
  - Gastrointestinal manometry
  - Defecography
- Diarrhea; if stool volume >400 mL/d:
  - Stool osmolarity and electrolytes
  - Jejunal aspirate for *Giardia lamblia*
  - Small-bowel and colon transit tests
  - Test rectal sensation
  - Cholestyramine
- Pain/gas/bloating:
  - Small-bowel x-ray
  - Trial of amitriptyline or other antidepressant
  - Carbohydrate H_2 breath test
  - Rectal sensation and emptying
  - Balloon dilatation test

6

Education and reassurance are particularly important with IBS. This should include an explanation that the intestine overreacts to a variety of stimuli and that this reaction may result in the symptoms described by the patient.

Treatment should be selected on the basis of (**Table 6.3**):

- Nature and severity of symptoms
- Degree of physiologic disturbance
- Effect of psychosocial difficulties.

It may be helpful to have patients monitor symptoms by keeping a diary for a period of time (eg, 2 to 3 weeks) to try to identify associated factors. This may open the door to changes in diet, lifestyle, or behavior that may be helpful. This also helps to provide a patient with a sense of greater control over the illness.

TABLE 6.3 — SEVERITY OF SYMPTOMS OF IRRITABLE BOWEL SYNDROME

Clinical Features	Mild	Moderate	Severe
Estimated prevalence	70%	25%	5%
Practice type	Primary	Specialty	Referral
Correlation with gut physiology*	Marked	Moderate	Mild
Symptoms constant	Generally absent	Mild	Marked
Psychosocial difficulties	Generally absent	Mild	Marked
Health care use	Mild	Moderate	Moderate

If mild symptoms: patient education, reassurance, dietary/lifestyle changes.

If moderate symptoms: gut-acting pharmacologic agents (anticholinergics, antidiarrheals, etc), psychological treatment in some cases.

If severe and refractory symptoms: antidepressant medication; mental health or pain-center referral may be needed.

* Symptoms are exacerbated by eating and relieved by defecation.

Dietary Modification

For the most part, specific food types are less important in the generation of symptoms than is the process of eating. However, foods that more commonly cause symptoms include:

- Fatty foods
- Beans and other gas-producing foods
- Alcohol
- Caffeine (may cause diarrhea)
- Lactose (in intolerant individuals)
- Excess fiber (in some people).

The patient should avoid an unnecessarily restrictive diet. Additionally, the patient should try to eliminate medications that may activate symptoms, ie, antacids and stimulant laxatives.

Dietary fiber is of controversial benefit in IBS. Control groups in some studies have similar degrees of improvement in symptoms. Symptom relief is not consistently associated with changes in bowel motility or stool weight.

A high-fiber diet is often utilized, especially in constipation-predominant patients. Unprocessed bran (such as Miller's Bran) can be used in increasing amounts up to 15 g/day until the desired effect is achieved. Hydrophilic colloids may be effective for both constipation and diarrhea. Taken with meals, hydrophilic colloids will help the patient retain water in stools, preventing both dehydration of stools and excessive water in the stools. They include:

- Psyllium compounds: Metamucil, Konsyl, Perdiem
- Carbophil compounds (may cause less gas and bloating): Citrucel powder, FiberCon tablets, Equalactin chewable tablets.

Additional dietary advice for patients with suspected IBS includes:
- Eating slowly
- Avoiding chewing gum and carbonated beverages
- Avoiding artificial sweeteners such as sorbitol (in sugar-free candies) and fructose.

Psychological Therapy

Many patients with IBS will benefit from clinical counseling. This type of intervention is potentially effective in patients whose symptoms are exacerbated or triggered by stress or if symptoms result in psychological distress and impaired quality of life. Counseling in addition to physiologically appropriate medication can bring relief to a subset of IBS patients.

Types of psychological treatments studied in IBS include:
- Cognitive-behavioral treatment
- Hypnosis
- Psychodynamic or interpersonal psychotherapy
- Relaxation/stress-management treatment.

Counseling is valuable in reducing anxiety and other psychological symptoms and often results in a reduction of gastrointestinal (GI) symptoms (especially abdominal pain and diarrhea), although it is unknown whether this is due to changes in GI physiology or to interpretation of enteroreceptive sensations. Patients more likely to respond to counseling are those:
- Who relate GI symptoms to life stresses
- With more typical IBS symptoms rather than chronic pain
- Younger than 50 years of age
- With a lesser degree of endogenous anxiety.

There are multidisciplinary pain-management programs that may help some patients with refractory pain associated with IBS. The focus is on behavioral strategies to increase symptom control. Anxiety and depression, provoked by chronic pain, may respond well. Such an approach is necessary only in a small minority of IBS patients.

Pharmacotherapy

Pharmacotherapy for IBS is targeted at specific symptoms such as:
- Abdominal pain and bloating
- Constipation
- Diarrhea.

■ Abdominal Pain and Bloating

Antispasmodics may be used to relieve the symptoms of abdominal pain and bloating. Anticholinergics block acetylcholine-mediated depolarization of intestinal smooth muscle. They include:
- Dicyclomine (Bentyl): 20 to 40 mg po qid
- Donnatal Extentabs— time-release, balanced combination antispasmodic with mild calming effect. Effective relief of cramping and diarrhea; well tolerated:
  - Dosage: 1 Extentab po bid or tid. Contains 0.3111 mg hyoscyamine, 0.0582 mg atropine, 0.0195 mg scopolamine and 48.6 mg phenobarbital
  - Extentabs are designed to release the ingredients gradually to provide effects for up to 12 hours
- Donnatal tablets and elixir (belladonna alkaloids with phenobarbital), 1 or 2 tablets (or 5 to 10 mL of elixir) po tid or qid

- Hyoscyamine (Levsin)—rapid onset of action helpful in relieving acute symptoms; results in reduced sigmoid motility after a fatty meal:
  - Oral/sublingual preparation: 0.125 mg po tid, or 1 to 2 tablets sublingually for acute abdominal pain due to spasm
  - Time-release formulation (Levbid): 0.375 mg po bid
  - Orally disintegrating 0.125 mg tablet (NuLev): 1 to 2 tablets allowed to dissolve on the tongue every 4 hours prn
- Librax (chlordiazepoxide plus clidinium bromide): 1 or 2 capsules before meals and at bedtime; withdrawal symptoms are possible with use of chlordiazepoxide.

The use of anticholinergics in treating IBS may be more effective than placebo in improving the patient's global assessment of well-being and decreasing abdominal pain.

■ **Constipation**

Increased dietary soluble fiber or psyllium products are often recommended. The possible beneficial effects of fiber include:
- Decreased whole-gut transit time
- Decreased intracolonic pressure, which may reduce pain
- Dilution of bile salts, which could indirectly reduce colonic contractile activity.

Tegaserod (Zelnorm) is a 5-hydroxytryptamine-4 (5-HT$_4$) receptor partial agonist that has been approved by the Food and Drug Administration (FDA) for use in women with constipation-predominant IBS. It is prescribed at a dosage of 6 mg po bid, although a starting dosage of 6 mg po once daily may be preferable for several days. A dosage of 2 mg po bid is recommended for patients with upper GI symptoms such as nonulcer dyspepsia, but the higher dose provides more consistent control of prominent colonic symptoms over time. It is currently recommended that it be prescribed for 4 to 6 weeks; then, if there is a positive response, it can be renewed for the same period of time.

It has been shown that serotonin (5-HT) plays a significant role in overall GI motility by way of its type-4 receptors. Most patients experience symptom relief within 1 to 2 weeks of the start of therapy. Stimulation of 5-HT_4 receptors triggers motor activity throughout the GI tract, particularly peristalsis, and also may suppress the visceral hypersensitivity to stimuli that plays a prominent role in the etiology of symptoms in IBS. In constipation-predominant IBS, tegaserod has demonstrated excellent relief of:

- Abdominal pain/discomfort
- Bloating
- Constipation (infrequent stools)
- Hard consistency of stools.

In placebo-controlled trials, each of these symptoms was relieved more effectively with tegaserod than by control to a statistically significant extent (**Figure 6.1**). Diarrhea occurred twice as frequently in patients using tegaserod compared with patients using placebo, however this most often occurred within the first week of treatment and usually did not require discontinuation of treatment. Side effects, particularly abdominal pain, diarrhea, flatulence, and headache, are no more frequent than with placebo, and specifically tegaserod has no demonstrable effect on the electrocardiogram. This is as opposed to a mixed serotonin agonist/5-HT_3 antagonist that was withdrawn from the market because of cardiac dysrhythmias. A few more patients taking tegaserod rather than placebo required

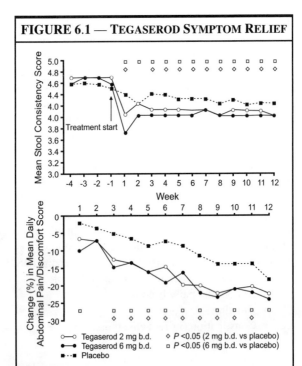

FIGURE 6.1 — TEGASEROD SYMPTOM RELIEF

Effect of tegaserod on the weekly stool consistency score *(top)*. Change from baseline in the severity of daily abdominal pain and discomfort *(bottom)*.

Müller-Lissner SA, et al. *Aliment Pharmacol Ther*. 2001;15: 1655-1666.

abdominal surgery (most often cholecystectomy), but a causal relationship with the medication has not been established. Phase III comparisons of tegaserod with standard therapy (fiber and antispasmodic medication) have not yet been carried out, but at the present time this is the only medication that is FDA-approved for constipation in patients with IBS.

■ Diarrhea

Pharmacologic agents used for controlling diarrhea associated with IBS include:

- Loperamide (Imodium), an opioid, 2 to 4 mg per dose, up to 16 mg/day:
  - Decreases colonic propulsive activity and transit
  - Enhances intestinal water and ion absorption
  - Strengthens anal sphincter tone, thereby improving diarrhea, urgency, and fecal soiling
  - Preferred over diphenoxylate, codeine, or other narcotics since it does not cross the blood-brain barrier
- Diphenoxylate plus atropine (Lomotil): 2 tablets or 10 mL of elixir po qid is recommended for treatment of acute diarrhea, but much smaller doses may be effective in some patients with diarrhea-predominant IBS. Diphenoxylate is the active ingredient and a subtherapeutic dose of atropine is added to discourage overdosage by causing anticholinergic side effects
- Cholestyramine (Questran powder), a chloride salt of a basic anion-exchange resin, in dosages of 1 to 2 packages or scoopfuls po bid:
  - Useful as a second-choice agent in patients with idiopathic bile acid malabsorption
  - Since bile acid malabsorption is often due to rapid transit, loperamide may be a more acceptable approach
  - Has a side effect of mild constipation
- Alosetron (Lotronex): 5-hydroxytryptamine-3 ($5HT_3$ or serotonin receptor antagonist); the only FDA-approved drug for patients with diarrhea-predominant IBS. Dosage is 1 mg po daily; if inadequate response at 4 weeks but no adverse reaction is reported, the dose can be increased to 1 mg po bid. Previously taken off

the market because of suspected ischemic colitis and other complications of severe constipation, it is now again available on a very restricted basis for women with IBS-related diarrhea if they have failed to respond to conventional therapy.

Although not specifically indicated for this use, low doses of certain antidepressant medications may be effective in some patients with severe refractory symptoms of IBS (**Table 6.4**). Tricyclic agents (eg, amitriptyline, imipramine, doxepin) and selective serotonin reuptake inhibitors (SSRIs) (eg, fluoxetine, sertraline, paroxetine) are used in some patients with IBS. The value of antidepressants may be related to the anticholinergic, antispasmodic, and analgesic effects of the medication. Antidepressant medications may:

- Improve the sleep cycle and overall sense of well-being
- Be helpful in IBS patients who have panic disorders or major depression
- Help improve GI symptoms sooner and with lower doses than expected when used for treatment of depression.

The effectiveness of antidepressant medications in the treatment of IBS requires chronic continuous use; thus they must be used selectively in patients with chronic or recurrent symptoms. Pain and diarrhea appear to be responsive to antidepressants, although SSRIs may prove more useful in patients with constipation-predominant IBS since a side effect of SSRIs is diarrhea. In general, SSRIs cause side effects less frequently than do tricyclic antidepressants at typical therapeutic doses.

A therapeutic trial of antidepressants should be used for at least 3 to 4 weeks at up to therapeutic doses

TABLE 6.4 — MAJOR ANTIDEPRESSANTS USED IN IRRITABLE BOWEL SYNDROME

Drug	Class	Dosage for Depression (mg/d)	Dosage for IBS (mg/d)	Side Effects
Amitriptyline	TCA	100-300	10-100	Co, S, X
Desipramine	TCA	100-300	10-200	Co, S, X
Fluoxetine	SSRI	10-20	10-20	D, Cr, N, A
Imipramine	TCA	100-300	10-100	Co, S, X
Paroxetine	SSRI	10-20	10-20	D, Cr, N, A
Sertraline	SSRI	50	50	D, Cr, N, A
Trazodone	Atypical	150-200	20-150	S, Co

Abbreviations: A, anxiety; Co, constipation; Cr, cramping; D, diarrhea; IBS, irritable bowel syndrome; N, nausea and vomiting; S, sedation; SSRI, selective serotonin reuptake inhibitor; TCA, tricyclic antidepressant; X, xerostomia.

and, if effective, for 3 to 12 months before tapering the dose. Adverse reactions are fairly unusual because of the low doses employed. Side effects of tricyclic antidepressants include constipation and xerostomia. Side effects of SSRIs include cramping and diarrhea (by stimulating intestinal motility) and, infrequently, nausea and vomiting.

Anxiolytics may be helpful in a minority of patients who experience a great deal of anxiety, but drug interactions and equivocal efficacy in IBS make benzodiazepines (eg, diazepam, lorazepam) less desirable.

SUGGESTED READING

American College of Gastroenterology Functional Gastrointestinal Disorders Task Force. Evidence-based position statement on the management of irritable bowel syndrome in North America. *Am J Gastroenterol.* 2002;97(suppl 11):S1-S5.

Camilleri M. Management of the irritable bowel syndrome. *Gastroenterology.* 2001;120:652-668.

Jackson JL, O'Malley PG, Tomkins G, Balden E, Santoro J, Kroenke K. Treatment of functional gastrointestinal disorders with antidepressant medications: a meta-analysis. *Am J Med.* 2000;108:65-72.

7 Diverticulosis and Acute Lower GI Bleeding

Diverticular disease of the colon or diverticulosis is defined as one or more areas of herniation of the colonic mucosa through the muscle layer of the colonic wall. Diverticulosis is unusual in patients under the age of 40 years, but the frequency increases with advancing age. There is a 35% to 50% prevalence of this disease in the general Western population, with a female-to-male ratio of 3:2. The average age of affected patients is 62 years, and more than 92% of people with diverticulosis are over the age of 50 years.

Diverticular disease is less common in South America and is rare in Africa and the Orient due to the higher vegetable and fiber intake of people in those areas. The sigmoid colon is involved in 95% to 97% of cases of diverticulosis in Western countries and is the only part of the colon affected in 65%. In Asian populations, it is usually localized to the right colon.

The prevalence of diverticulosis according to age is as follows:
- <5% at age 40
- 30% at 60 years
- 65% at 85 years
- 80% at age >85 years.

Pathogenesis

Most colonic diverticula are acquired and are actually pseudodiverticula, which represent herniation of only the mucosa through the muscular wall of the colon. True diverticula, with herniation of all layers of the bowel wall, are congenital lesions that rarely occur in the colon, except occasionally in the cecum.

The colon has an outer longitudinal muscular coat that forms three longitudinal strips, the taeniae coli, and an inner circular muscle surrounding the submucosa as a single layer. The outer muscular wall is weakest at the points where the vasa recta of the colonic wall penetrate from the muscularis into the submucosa. Diverticula most often form at these points and usually include an arterial branch of the vasa recta, which may be related to the pathophysiology of diverticular bleeding.

A common mechanism of the development of diverticula in the descending and sigmoid colon is that the colonic wall in some affected patients is redundant, with thickening of both the longitudinal and circular muscle layers. This results in a shortening of the taeniae (or so-called *myochosis*), which may narrow the colonic lumen and can cause pericolic fibrosis. When these contractions obliterate the lumen, the increased pressure in compressed segments facilitates diverticulum formation.

A diet low in fiber decreases the volume and weight of stool present in the colon. Teleologically, it is believed that muscular hypertrophy develops in an effort to transport the small amount of material through the colon. The resultant intraluminal hypertension allows diverticula to form when the mucosa herniates through the muscularis of the colonic wall. This process is detailed in **Figures 7.1 and 7.2**.

Clinical Patterns of Diverticular Disease

Most commonly, diverticular disease is asymptomatic. Diverticulosis may be an incidental finding with barium enema, computed tomography (CT) scan,

FIGURE 7.1 — SCHEMATIC DEMONSTRATION OF THE DEVELOPMENT OF DIVERTICULA

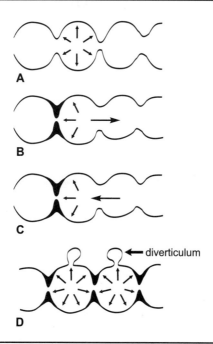

(A) Contraction of a single colonic segment results in increased intraluminal pressure. (B) Relaxation at one end of a segment during contraction allows fecal matter to be transported distally along the lumen. (C) Failure to relax at one end of a chamber can reduce or even halt transit of intestinal contents along the lumen. (D) Complete isolation of one or more segments during contraction causes dramatic increases in intraluminal pressure, thereby predisposing to diverticulum formation.

Adapted from: Painter NS. *Ann R Coll Surg*. 1964;34:111.

7

FIGURE 7.2 — SCHEMATIC DEMONSTRATION OF THE RELATION OF DIVERTICULUM TO COLONIC VESSELS

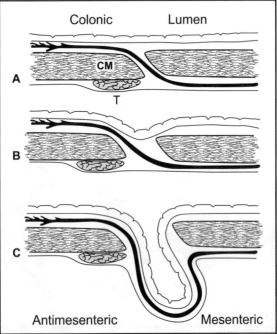

(A) The vasa recta penetrates the colonic wall at specific sites in the circular muscle (CM), usually along the mesenteric side of the taeniae (T). (B) As a diverticulum begins to herniate through the colonic wall, the blood vessels are drawn along. (C) The vasa recta eventually become draped over the dome of the diverticulum and are prone to rupture after trauma from within the lumen of the colon.

Adapted from: Meyers MA, et al. *Gastroenterology*. 1976;71: 577.

colonoscopy, or sigmoidoscopy with no attributable symptoms.

Painful diverticular disease occurs with chronic localized abdominal pain with no other organic abnormalities (intestinal, gynecologic, or genitourinary), except for diverticulosis.

Bleeding may occur from a diverticulum, or diverticulitis may result from either a localized or a free perforation.

Clinical Manifestations

Most patients with diverticular disease have either no symptoms or only minor symptoms. Symptoms may be nonspecific, such as:

- Intermittent abdominal pain
- Bloating
- Excessive flatulence
- Irregular defecation
- Pellet-like stools or diarrhea.

Narrow-caliber stools or rectal bleeding should be evaluated to rule out carcinoma, which shares the features of diverticulosis in being more common in older age and often affecting the left colon. Narrow stools in the presence of diverticulosis and without cancer may alternatively be due to coexisting spasm from the irritable bowel syndrome (IBS) or from stricturing after repeated episodes of diverticulitis.

Diagnosis

The barium enema is useful in diagnosing other conditions that may be clinically mimicked or masked by diverticulosis. It is the test of choice for documenting the number and extent of diverticula, but possibly because of tortuosity and overlap of segments of the sigmoid colon, it may be suboptimal in ruling out concomitant conditions such as colitis or cancer. The barium enema may show barium retained in diverticula, spasm, or sacculation of the colonic wall.

A CT scan can document the presence of diverticula. It reveals the colonic lumen and the wall poorly, however.

Sigmoidoscopy or colonoscopy will readily demonstrate the presence of diverticular orifices and may infrequently document that bleeding is attributable to diverticulosis. However, these endoscopic procedures are best utilitized for evaluating the colon for other conditions such as colitis or cancer in patients with symptoms of bleeding or nonspecific symptoms that may be suggestive of partial or intermittent colonic obstruction. Endoscopy should always be used in the evaluation of significant lower gastrointestinal (GI) bleeding unless contraindicated for other reasons. If tortuosity or stricturing prevents passage of a colonoscope and a clear diagnosis cannot be made, surgical resection should be seriously considered.

Painful Diverticular Disease

Chronic abdominal pain attributable to intense colonic muscle contractions and resultant colonic luminal hypertension may occur in the absence of diverticulitis. A tender palpable sigmoid colon may be noted upon physical examination. Painful diverticular disease may be difficult to distinguish from IBS. An attempt should be made to manage this problem with a high-fiber diet, as can be used in IBS.

Lower Gastrointestinal Bleeding/ Diverticular Bleeding

Diverticular bleeding occurs in 15% to 40% of patients with diverticulosis and may be massive in 5%

of those patients. This is the most common cause of massive lower GI bleeding in adults and accounts for 30% to 50% of such cases. However, it is exceedingly difficult to document that diverticula are responsible for bleeding, causing this to often be a diagnosis of exclusion.

In suspected diverticular bleeding, colonoscopy should be performed to look for other treatable causes of lower GI bleeding such as:

- Arteriovenous malformation (AVM)
- Colitis:
  - Inflammatory bowel disease
  - Ischemic colitis
  - Infectious colitis
- Adenomatous polyps
- Cancer.

Severe colonic bleeding most often occurs in the right colon, where AVMs are usually seen and where up to 90% of diverticular bleeding occurs, presumably because the wall of the right colon is much thinner than that of the left colon. Diverticular bleeding is usually the result of injury to the arterial vasa recta in a diverticulum. Local inflammation (diverticulitis) is typically not present. The risk of rebleeding after a diverticular bleeding incident is 30% after the first episode and 50% after a second episode.

■ Management of Uncomplicated Diverticulosis

The mainstay of treatment of patients with either asymptomatic or uncomplicated diverticular disease is to add fiber to the diet. Fiber serves to increase stool weight (bulk), lower colonic pressure, and increase transit time, all of which may prevent muscular thickening and resultant intraluminal hypertension that may perpetuate or exacerbate symptoms of diverticulosis.

■ Initial Patient Care in Major Acute Lower Gastrointestinal Bleeding

A large-bore intravenous access should be inserted promptly for hydration. A nasogastric tube should be passed to rule out an upper GI source of bleeding. A catheter should be used to monitor urinary output. Blood is drawn for type and crossmatch, a complete blood count, coagulation studies (prothrombin time, partial thromboplastin time), and other studies, if indicated.

■ Diagnostic Studies in Acute Lower Gastrointestinal Bleeding

Proctoscopy

An algorithm of the evaluation of acute lower GI bleeding is shown in **Figure 7.3**. Proctoscopy or flexible sigmoidoscopy should be done promptly in all cases of massive lower GI bleeding in the event that emergency subtotal colectomy needs to be considered in an exsanguinating bleed. Internal hemorrhoids and rectal disease should be excluded before an extensive colectomy is done unnecessarily.

Nuclear Scanning

Nuclear scanning with ^{99m}Tc sulfur colloid and ^{99m}Tc-tagged red blood cells is a very sensitive study, requiring only 0.1 mL/min bleeding for positivity. Repeated scanning over 24 to 36 hours after injection of isotope may be useful in cases of intermittent bleeding. It is a nonspecific test, but it is useful as a screening test to approximate the location of the bleeding site before a more definitive test such as angiography or colonoscopy is done.

Angiography

Angiography is the test of choice when brisk bleeding occurs. It is a sensitive and specific procedure if at least 0.5 mL/min bleeding is occurring. It

FIGURE 7.3 — ALGORITHM FOR LOWER GASTROINTESTINAL BLEEDING

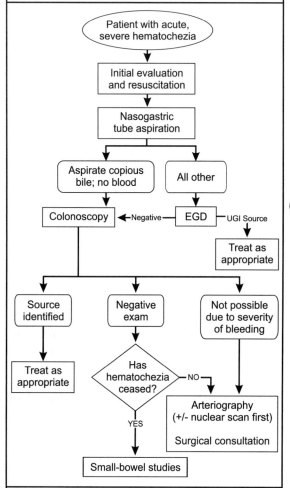

Abbreviations: EGD, esophagogastroduodenoscopy; UGI, upper gastrointestinal (tract).

Adapted from: Zuccaro G Jr. *Am J Gastroenterol.* 1998:93; 1202-1208.

may show extravasation of arterially infused contrast in a pattern typical of tumor, colitis, or angiodysplasia.

The arterial blood supply of the colon is shown in **Figure 7.4**. The superior mesenteric artery (SMA) delivers blood to the proximal transverse colon, the ascending colon, and the cecum (and much of the small intestine). The inferior mesenteric artery (IMA) serves the distal transverse colon down to the rectum. If the area of bleeding is unknown, the SMA should be injected first and the IMA should be injected next. If necessary, the celiac artery can be injected in order to examine the upper GI tract.

Examination of the SMA and the IMA will be diagnostic in 70% to 100% of cases of ongoing bleeding. Diagnostic accuracy is best if angiography is reserved for patients with a positive nuclear bleeding scan.

One angiographic therapeutic option in active colonic bleeding is placement of a catheter for intra-arterial infusion of the vasoconstrictor vasopressin, which controls active bleeding in more than 90% of cases. Vasopressin intra-arterial infusion can be started at 0.1 to 0.2 U/min. If bleeding continues, the infusion is increased to a maximum of 0.4 U/min. If bleeding then ceases, the infusion is continued for an additional 24 hours. There is a high risk of rebleeding (> 50%), however, when vasopressin is discontinued.

Angiographic embolization can be performed with autologous blood, Gelfoam or metal microcoils. Thrombogenesis due to injection of one of these substances will occlude the vessel, eliminating continued bleeding. Gelfoam breaks into small particles and may be carried out to very small vascular branches, resulting in a significant risk of colonic infarction. A larger, thicker coil that impacts in a larger vessel is safer in that it may cause ischemia but is less likely to cause infarction. Coil embolization may eliminate the need for surgery in some cases or change an emergent sur-

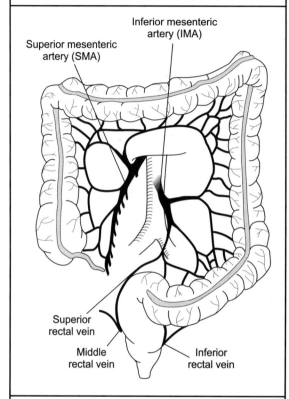

FIGURE 7.4 — ANATOMY AND BLOOD SUPPLY OF THE LARGE INTESTINE

Inferior mesenteric artery (IMA)

Superior mesenteric artery (SMA)

Superior rectal vein

Middle rectal vein

Inferior rectal vein

Adapted from: Beart RW Jr, Nivatvong S, Wolff B. The colon, rectum and anus. In: Nora PF, ed. *Operative Surgery*. 3rd ed. Philadelphia, Pa: WB Saunders Co; 1990.

gical procedure (with greater morbidity and mortality) into a safer elective operation. A coil may also serve to help the surgeon more easily localize the source of bleeding intraoperatively. Embolization may be preferable to vasopressin infusion when bleeding originates in a larger vessel, while vasopressin is less likely to cause significant ischemia or infarction in a more peripheral bleed from a smaller artery.

Colonoscopy

Colonoscopy is the diagnostic test of choice if lower GI bleeding appears to have stopped and is useful after a normal bleeding scan or if angiography is normal after a positive bleeding scan. Rapid preparation can be carried out over 2 to 4 hours using a colonic lavage of 4 L (ie, GoLYTELY or CoLYTE). There is, however, a small risk of congestive heart failure (4%) as a result of the large volume a patient must ingest to clear the colonic lumen.

Colonoscopy is diagnostic in 85% to 90% of cases with a nonbleeding lesion. While it is relatively uncommon to document definite diverticular bleeding, colonoscopic treatment with epinephrine injection, bipolar coagulation, or both, have good success in preventing rebleeding and are able to diminish the likelihood that surgery will be necessary.

SUGGESTED READING

Beart RW Jr, Nivatvong S, Wolff B. The colon, rectum and anus. In: Nora PF, ed. *Operative Surgery*. 3rd ed. Philadelphia, Pa: WB Saunders Co; 1990.

Jensen DM, Machicado GA, Jutabha R, Kovacs TO. Urgent colonoscopy for the diagnosis and treatment of severe diverticular hemorrhage. *N Engl J Med*. 2000;342:78-82.

Meyers MA, Alonso DR, Gray GF, Baer JW. Pathogenesis of bleeding colonic diverticulosis. *Gastroenterology*. 1976;71:577-583.

Painter NS. The aetiology of diverticulosis of the colon with special reference to the action of certain drugs on the behavior of the colon. *Ann R Coll Surg*. 1964;34:111.

Rolandelli RH, Roslyn JJ. Colon and rectum. In: Townsend CM, Beauchamp DR, Evers MB, et al, eds. *Sabiston Textbook of Surgery: The Bioloical Basis of Modern Surgical Practice*. 16th ed. Philadelphia, Pa: WB Saunders Co; 2001:929-973.

Zuccaro G Jr. Managment of the adult patient with acute lower gastrointestinal bleeding. American College of Gastroenterology. Practice Parameters Committee. *Am J Gastroenterol*. 1998;93:1202-1208.

7

8 Diverticulitis

Diverticulitis occurs when a diverticulum perforates and may result in more serious consequences. This complication occurs in 10% to 25% of patients with previously recognized diverticulosis. The risk of developing diverticulitis increases with time:

- 10% after 5 years with diverticulosis
- 35% after 20 years with diverticulosis.

Sixty percent of patients with a first episode of diverticulitis will have only mild illness and can be treated as outpatients with antibiotic therapy. The antibiotic regimen selected should treat infection caused by enterobacteriaceae, *Bacteroides* species, and, less frequently, *Pseudomonas aeruginosa* and enterococci. Diverticulitis almost always occurs in the sigmoid colon in patients in the United States.

Pathogenesis

Inspissated fecal matter in a diverticulum may form a fecalith. The fecalith causes impaction within the diverticulum and local mucosal inflammation ensues. Inflammation and ensuing necrosis progress to a microperforation or a macroperforation.

A microperforation is initially contained by pericolonic tissues such as mesentery, fat, or adjacent organs, resulting in an inflammatory mass or phlegmon. Repeated microperforations may result in more extensive phlegmon development and may lead to fibrosis of the colonic wall, creating a stricture or obstruction.

A macroperforation is the result of free perforation with generalized peritonitis. A peridiverticular abscess may be locally contained, or the septic process may erode into adjacent structures as a sinus tract or fistula.

Symptoms

Left lower-quadrant abdominal pain occurs in 93% to 100% of patients with diverticulitis, often associated with an alteration in bowel habits. Fever is seen in about 86% of patients; of this percentage of patients, half will experience only a low-grade fever. If a fistula to the urinary tract has developed, the patient may experience frequency, urgency, pneumaturia, or fecaluria. Leukocytosis is seen in 69% to 93% of patients.

Signs

Left lower-quadrant abdominal tenderness is the predominant sign of diverticulitis. The patient may also show clinical signs of peritonitis, experiencing hyperthermia and severe abdominal pain with rebound tenderness and involuntary guarding. A tender inflammatory mass (phlegmon) may be palpable. Jaundice may be seen in the rare complication of pylephlebitis.

The differential diagnosis of diverticulitis includes:

- Colon cancer
- Inflammatory bowel disease
- Painful diverticular disease without perforation
- Appendicitis (if pain is right-sided)
- Perforated peptic ulcer
- Irritable bowel syndrome.

Right Colonic Diverticulitis

A rare condition in Western countries, right colonic diverticulitis is most often identified at surgery when appendicitis is expected. Differences between right-sided diverticulitis and appendicitis are outlined in **Table 8.1**.

Initial Diagnostic Studies in Diverticulitis

A complete blood count should be drawn, looking for leukocytosis. A white blood cell count >15,000 should raise suspicion of an intra-abdominal abscess.

A urinalysis may demonstrate white blood cells if a phlegmon is adjacent to the bladder or ureters. If bacteria are present, a fistula should be suspected.

An obstruction series should be performed, with supine and upright abdominal x-rays. Subdiaphragmatic free air suggests a perforation. Retroperitoneal air may also be seen. A large abscess may cause a mass effect on the colon. Air-fluid levels may be seen if there is obstruction or an ileus. If the diagnosis is uncertain, additional radiographic studies are useful (**Table 8.2**).

Management of Uncomplicated Acute Diverticulitis

Decisions for treatment depend on the:
- Severity of the acute episode
- Pace of improvement
- Patient's age and immune status
- Presence or absence of right-sided diverticulosis.

In mild disease, treatment may include the following:
- Liquid or low-residue diet
- Oral antibiotics for 7 to 10 days. Possible oral antibiotic regimens include:
  - Metronidazole: 500 mg po every 6 hours with either:

TABLE 8.1 — DIFFERENCES BETWEEN RIGHT-SIDED DIVERTICULITIS AND APPENDICITIS		
	Diverticulitis	**Appendicitis**
Average age	44 years	Much younger
Duration of symptoms	3.3 days	24 hours
Location of symptoms	RLQ of abdomen only	Epigastrium initially, then to RLQ
Frequency of nausea	20%	80%
Abbreviation: RLQ, right lower quadrant.		

- Trimethoprim/sulfamethoxazole (Bactrim), 1 double-strength tablet po bid, or
- Ciprofloxacin (Cipro), 500 mg po bid
- Amoxicillin/clavulanate (Augmentin) (875/125 mg po bid or 500/125 mg po tid).

After the acute attack has resolved, the patient should consume a high-fiber diet (20 to 30 g fiber per day). A barium enema or colonoscopy should be performed in 4 to 6 weeks to rule out polyps or cancer. Vague symptoms such as crampy abdominal pain are reported after a first episode of diverticulitis by 30% to 40% of patients. Surgery is usually not indicated since only 20% to 30% of patients have a recurrence after a first episode. Recurrences usually take place within 5 years of the initial episode.

After a second or third episode, however, surgery should be considered 4 to 6 weeks after the inflammation has resolved. In this setting, 90% of patients have ongoing symptoms and 60% have complications. Each recurrent attack may be associated with greater morbidity and mortality than earlier episodes. Open or laparoscopic resection and primary anastomosis are usually curative.

Acute diverticulitis before the age of 40 years, even in the absence of immediate complications, is considered an indication for surgery in itself by many because of a much greater frequency of delayed complications.

Indications for hospitalization in acute diverticulitis include:
- Severe pain
- Inability to tolerate an oral diet
- Failure of symptoms to promptly resolve or worsening of symptoms with outpatient treatment
- Clinical toxicity (high fever, worsening leukocytosis).

TABLE 8.2 — DIAGNOSTIC OPTIONS IN ACUTE DIVERTICULITIS

Diagnostic Study	Diagnostic Findings	Advantage(s)	Disadvantage(s)
Computed tomography (CT) scan	• Inflamed pericolic fat • Presence of one or more diverticula • Colonic wall thickening • Evidence of a peridiverticular abscess (in colonic wall or mesocolon) • Ureteral obstruction (hydronephrosis or hydroureter) • Absence of evidence of other related diagnoses, such as cancer or inflammatory bowel disease	• The most cost-effective and safest diagnostic study, with therapeutic use in drainage of an abscess • Does not increase intraluminal pressure • Allows evaluation of pericolonic structures (ureters, distant sites of abscess formation) • Localizes abscesses and phlegmons • Can be used to follow resolution of inflammatory process	• Misses the diagnosis of diverticulitis in up to 20% of cases, when thickened colonic wall without abscess seen suggests cancer
Ultrasound	• Thickened hypoechoic colonic wall • Zone of hyperechogenicity surrounding the area of disease	• Noninvasive • Inexpensive • Readily and widely available	• Highly operator-dependent • Suboptimal image quality in obese patients or if great deal of gas is present

Ultrasound (cont.)	• Presence of one or more diverticula • Pain on compression of the affected segment	• Can be used therapeutically for abscess drainage	• Local tenderness may make it impossible to apply enough pressure to visualize diseased area of colon • May be inadequate to distinguish cancer from diverticulitis
Contrast enema (barium or Gastrograffin)	• Diverticula • Segmental sigmoid narrowing • Extravasation of contrast (due to perforation or fistulization)	• Demonstrates stenosis of lumen best	• Insufflation during examination may cause dislodgment of a fecalith and may result in perforation • Barium has the potential of causing a severe peritoneal reaction if there is extravasation. This can be avoided with a water-soluble enema such as Gastrograffin • The same findings can be demonstrated more safely with CT scan or ultrasound

8

Continued

Diagnostic Study	Diagnostic Findings	Advantage(s)	Disadvantage(s)
Colonoscopy/ sigmoidoscopy	• Diverticula • Resistance to passage of instrument due to stricturing or spasm • Peridiverticular inflammation or pus • Evidence of perforation or fistulization	• Effective means of excluding alternative explanations of symptoms, such as inflammatory bowel disease, infectious colitis, ischemic bowel disease, or cancer	• Relatively contraindicated in acute diverticulitis because of the risk of perforation • If needed, should be done with little pressure and with minimal air insufflation

In-hospital management should include:

- Nothing by mouth
- Intravenous (IV) hydration
- Nasogastric tube if there is significant nausea or vomiting
- Surgical consultation
- Frequent serial clinical assessment
- Intravenous antibiotics must cover aerobic and anaerobic gram-negative organisms as well as enterococci. The most common gram-negative organisms identified in diverticulitis are enterobacteriaceae such as *Escherichia coli*, *Bacteroides* species (particularly *B fragilis*), and, more so with ruptured diverticulitis, *Pseudomonas aeruginosa*. Effective antibiotic options include:
  - In mild-moderate diverticulitis requiring hospitalization:
    - Ampicillin/sulbactam: 3 mg IV every 6 hours or
    - Piperacillin/tazobactam: 3.375 g IV every 6 hours or 4.5 g IV every 8 hours or
    - Ticarcillin/clavulanate: 3.1 g IV every 6 hours or
    - Ertapenem 1 m IV daily
  - Severe life-threatening diverticulitis with diffuse peritonitis should be treated with:
    - Imipenem/cilastin 500 mg IV every 6 hours or
    - Meropenem 1 g IV every 8 hours or
    - Piperacillin/tazobactam: 3.375 g IV every 6 hours or 4.5 g IV every 8 hours or
    - Ampicillin 1 to 2 g IV every 4 to 6 hours plus gentamicin 1.5 to 2 mg/kg IV every 8 hours plus metronidazole 500 mg IV every 8 hours.

When parenteral analgesia is required, meperidine (Demerol) is effective and well tolerated. Morphine should be avoided as it may precipitate or exacerbate colonic spasm. A computed tomography (CT) scan should be ordered or repeated in 48 to 72 hours if symptoms worsen or if there is no improvement in order to look for complications (free perforation or abscess). Surgery should be considered in this setting.

If the patient is improving in the hospital, oral antibiotics can be completed at home for a total of 7 to 10 days. The patient can be advanced to a low-fiber diet as tolerated.

Complications of Diverticulitis

■ **Fistulas**

The most common fistula encountered as a complication of diverticulitis is colovesical, between the colon and urinary bladder. Causes of a colovesical fistula include:

- Diverticulitis (52%)
- Crohn's disease (18%)
- Carcinoma (11%)
- Other malignancy.

This fistula is far more common in men than in women, with a raio up to 6:1. Most women affected (83%) have undergone hysterectomy (since the uterus lies between the sigmoid colon and the bladder). Signs and symptoms may include:

- Dysuria (29% to 94%)
- Fecaluria (50% to 75%)
- Pneumaturia (air in the urinary tract) (40% to 75%)
- Abdominal pain or signs of systemic infection (25% to 30%)
- Symptoms of urinary tract infection (75%).

Diagnosis of a colovesical fistula may include:
- CT scan (demonstrates air in the bladder)
- Colonoscopy:
  - To rule out sigmoid carcinoma, which requires wider surgical resection
  - To assess extent and severity of inflammatory reaction
  - Can document a fistula 20% of the time
- Barium enema:
  - Documents the presence of diverticulosis
  - Demonstrates the fistula 50% of the time
- Cystogram or cystoscopy:
  - Fistulous opening seen in 50%
  - Bullous edema or localized cystitis seen in 90%.

Management of colovesical fistulas includes the treatment of the underlying sepsis as the first priority. If urosepsis occurs, the bladder should be drained with a urethral or suprapubic catheter and parenteral antibiotics administered. Emergent surgery is rarely needed. After initial care, the colon can usually be adequately prepared to perform a one-step colonic resection with primary anastomosis (possible in 90% of cases). A bladder resection is usually unnecessary in the management of a colovesical fistula.

Colocutaneous fistulas virtually only occur after surgery for diverticulitis; only 5% occur spontaneously. Treatment involves sigmoidectomy, possible omental interposition, and (in women) possible closure of the vaginal apex.

With a coloenteric fistula, colonic resection is usually required. A small-bowel resection with primary reanastomosis is needed only if the affected area is indurated or obviously inflamed. Less common are fistulas to the ureter, uterus, fallopian tubes, perineum, and the venous system.

■ Abscesses

Abscesses are the most common complication of sigmoid diverticulitis and are the result of diverticular perforation. Abscesses should be suspected if diverticulitis does not improve after 48 to 72 hours of appropriate treatment.

For a localized abscess that is contained in or adjacent to the colonic wall, the physical findings include abdominal tenderness, fullness, or a mass. There may be localized peritoneal signs and tachycardia. A CT scan can provide the diagnosis and may allow percutaneous drainage to be performed. Treatment includes bowel rest and broad-spectrum antibiotics. Percutaneous drainage can reduce subsequent surgery to a one-step procedure in up to 80% of patients, and in patients who cannot tolerate surgery, it may be adequate to relieve symptoms.

A pelvic abscess may occur when diverticular perforation is contained by adjacent pelvic structures. Clinical presentation is similar to that of a localized abscess. Rectal or vaginal examination may reveal a tender bulging mass. Management is the same as for a localized abscess. Options include transrectal or transvaginal drainage guided by ultrasound through the rectum or vaginal wall, respectively.

Distant abscesses may rarely be found in the liver, hip, thigh, abdominal wall, or other locations. Percutaneous drainage, guided by CT or ultrasound, can be performed; when done preoperatively, this may permit a simpler subsequent surgical procedure to be performed. Drainage of peridiverticular abscesses should be restricted to large collections (>5 cm in diameter) as smaller abscesses often regress with antibiotics alone. If the abscess cavity contains feculent material, prompt surgical intervention is required to control sepsis.

■ Generalized Peritonitis

Generalized peritonitis occurs when a free perforation from diverticulitis occurs in the peritoneal cavity. Overall mortality is 20% to 40%, usually due to septic shock and multiorgan system failure. The peritonitis can be purulent or feculent.

Purulent peritonitis occurs with sudden rupture of a walled-off abscess or from continued leakage at the diverticular perforation. Obstruction of the diverticulum by a fecalith protects against gross fecal peritonitis. Signs and symptoms include:

- Severe abdominal pain
- Tenderness with voluntary or involuntary guarding
- Intraperitoneal free air (seen often but not always)
- Leukocytosis with a left shift (though leukopenia may occur if patient is septic, elderly, or immunocompromised).

Broad-spectrum antibiotics are given, and surgical resected specimen should be opened and cancer ruled out before closure of abdomen. An end-descending colostomy is usually created. The mortality rate in this setting is 6%.

Feculent peritonitis is the most dangerous complication of diverticulitis, with a 35% mortality rate. It is usually due to rupture of an uninflamed diverticulum. There is leakage of fecal material into the peritoneal space. An emergency colostomy is necessary and, if possible, is accompanied by resection of the diseased segment.

Indications for Surgery in Acute Diverticulitis

Indications for immediate surgery include:
- Complications of diverticulitis:
  - Intractable or recurrent hemorrhage
  - Sepsis (abscess, generalized peritonitis)
  - Obstruction
- Recurrent episodes of inflammation
- Intractable symptoms or signs (persistent pain or mass)
- Clinical deterioration despite maximal medical therapy
- Inability to exclude carcinoma, especially in an immunocompromised patient
- Massively dilated cecum (to >10 cm)
- Signs of cecal necrosis (eg, air in bowel wall)
- Marked right lower-quadrant tenderness in presence of a dilated cecum
- Generalized peritonitis
- Visceral perforation.

Indications for elective surgery include:
- Chronic stricture
- Fistula formation
- Recurrent diverticulitis
- Patient who concurrently requires corticosteroid medication for a separate chronic condition
- Any patient under the age of 40 (controversial).

Surgical Management of Acute Diverticulitis

In any surgical procedure for sigmoid diverticulitis, the rectosigmoid junction should be resected in addition to sigmoidectomy to avoid recurrence. All of the colon with thickened muscular walls should be resected and not necessarily the entire segment containing diverticula. Laparoscopy can be used for sigmoid resection in some elective cases.

■ Surgical Options
One-Step Procedure

Sigmoid resection and primary colocolic anastomosis is the most common operation performed if preoperative bowel preparation is possible. It is the operation of choice in uncomplicated diverticulitis. It also can be used if an abscess has been drained preoperatively, even in the presence of a fistula.

This procedure is contraindicated if there is significant intra-abdominal infection or if the more proximal areas of the colon cannot be adequately prepared preoperatively.

Two-Step Hartmann's Procedure

This procedure is used in the emergency treatment of diverticulitis. The first step is resection with sigmoid colostomy and closure of the rectal stump, thereby removing the source of ongoing infection. The second step, performed 3 to 6 months later, includes takedown of the colostomy and reestablishment of bowel continuity with a colorectal anastomosis.

SUGGESTED READING

Cunningham MA, Davis JW, Kaups KL. Medical versus surgical management of diverticulitis in patients under age 40. *Am J Surg*. 1997;174:733-736.

Ferzoco LB, Raptopoulos V, Silen W. Acute diverticulitis. *N Engl J Med*. 1998;338:1521-1526.

Gilbert DN, Moellering RC, Sande MA. *The Sanford Guide to Antimicrobial Therapy 2003*. 33rd ed. Hyde Park, Vt: Antimicrobial Therapy, Inc; 2003.

Imbembo AL. Diverticular disease of the colon. In: Sabiston DC. *Textbook of Surgery: The Biological Basis of Modern Surgical Practice*. 14th ed. Philadelphia, Pa: WB Saunders; 1991.

9 IBD: General Information

Inflammatory bowel disease (IBD) is comprised of two related conditions:
- Ulcerative colitis (UC)
- Crohn's disease.

These are chronic conditions of the digestive tract. While UC is limited to the rectum and colon, Crohn's disease may be present anywhere in the entire gastrointestinal tract. **Table 9.1** shows some of the clinical similarities and differences between these two diseases.

Etiology

There is a great deal of evidence suggesting that susceptibility to IBD (particularly Crohn's disease) has a genetic basis. With the use of microsatellite DNA markers, it has been shown that some families with several relatives affected with Crohn's disease have an abnormal locus on chromosome 16 called IBD1. Linkage to several other genomic regions has been associated with both common forms of IBD. A gene on chromosome 16 produces a protein gene product called NOD2 or CARD 15 (caspase activation and recruitment domain), variants of which appear to confer a substantially increased risk of developing Crohn's disease.

Factors other than genetics also play a role in the development of IBD. These include:
- Nonsteroidal anti-inflammatory drug use, which may precipitate IBD flares
- Appendectomy before the age of 20 years, which appears to be protective against the development of ulcerative colitis

TABLE 9.1 — KEY FEATURES OF MAJOR FORMS OF INFLAMMATORY BOWEL DISEASE		
Feature	Ulcerative Colitis	Crohn's Disease
Clinical Features		
Fever	Fairly common	Common
Abdominal pain	Varies	Common
Diarrhea	Very common	Fairly common
Rectal bleeding	Very common	Fairly common
Weight loss	Fairly common	Common
Signs of malnutrition	Fairly common	Common
Perianal disease	Absent	Fairly common
Abdominal mass	Absent	Common
Growth failure in children and adolescents	Occasional	Common
Site		
Colon	Exclusively	Two thirds of patients
Ileum	Never	Two thirds of patients
Jejunum	Never	Infrequent
Stomach or duodenum	Never	Infrequent
Esophagus	Never	Infrequent

Intestinal Complications		
Stricture	Unknown	Common
Fistulas	Absent	Fairly common
Toxic megacolon	Unknown	Absent
Perforation	Unknown	Uncommon
Cancer	Common	Fairly common
Endoscopic Findings		
Friability	Very common	Fairly common
Aphthous and linear ulcers	Absent	Common
Cobblestone appearance	Absent	Common
Pseudopolyps	Common	Fairly common
Rectal involvement	Very common	Fairly common
Radiologic Findings		
Distribution	Continuous	Discontinuous, segmented
Ulceration	Fine, superficial	Deep, with submucosal extension
Fissures	Absent	Common
Strictures of fistulas	Rare	Common
Ileal involvement	Dilated ("backwash ileitis")	Narrowed, nodular

Continued

9

123

Feature	Ulcerative Colitis	Crohn's Disease
Laboratory Findings		
Perinuclear-staining antineutrophil cytoplasmic antibodies	70% of patients	Occasional
Anti–*Saccharomyces cerevisiae* antibodies	Occasional	>50% of patients

Podalsky DK. Inflammatory bowel disease. *N Engl J Med.* 2002;347:419.

- Smoking, which appears to increase the risk of Crohn's disease while decreasing the risk of UC
- Surface-adherent and intracellular colonic bacteria are increased in number in some patients with IBD, motivating the use of broad-spectrum antibiotics and probiotics in some such patients.

Certain subtypes of lymphocytes produce inflammatory cytokines (various interleukins, macrophage migration inhibitor factor, tumor necrosis factor [TNF]), chemokines, growth factors, arachidonic acid metabolites, and metabolites of reactive oxygen species and are predominant in IBD patients. These factors contribute to the inflammatory process and to tissue destruction.

Management

The inflammatory manifestations of UC and Crohn's disease are treated with a similar array of medications. Milder disease is often treated with orally or rectally administered aminosalicylates, chemically related to aspirin, which serve a topical anti-inflammatory function when released in affected areas of the intestinal tract. Disease refractory to aminosalicylates can be treated acutely with corticosteroids, while maintenance of remission may require immunomodulatory or immunosuppressive agents, either alone or in combination with aminosalicylates. Antibiotics have a role in the management of perianal fistulae and perineal involvement in Crohn's disease. Newer approaches to therapy include:
- Nonsystemic corticosteroids
- Fish oils
- Monoclonal antibodies.

Enteral and parenteral nutritional support plays an important adjunctive role in the management of IBD, which is frequently complicated by malnutrition. Supplemental nutrition may obviate the need for hospitalization or surgery by allowing some patients the time to achieve optimal benefit from medication. Others will tolerate surgery more easily by entering the operating room in a better nourished state.

Surgery plays a very different role in UC than it does in Crohn's disease. When medically refractory colitis or a complication of UC necessitates surgery, most patients will undergo a total proctocolectomy. Not only does this operation cure the underlying disease, but it eliminates the substantial cancer risk that exists after having UC for several years. In Crohn's disease, surgery cannot be curative and is reserved for situations in which medication is either ineffective or intolerable or if a complication develops that cannot be treated otherwise. The goal of surgery in this condition is to resolve the acute situation, restore a better quality of life, and simplify the medical regimen.

Anastomotic lines from bowel resection are at an especially high risk of recurrent Crohn's disease. Surgical options are discussed separately in the following chapters.

Nutrition

Malnutrition and weight loss are identified in more than half of hospitalized IBD patients. Reasons for weight loss include:
- Poor oral intake
- Increased nutrient losses due to vomiting or diarrhea
- Malabsorption
- Increased nutritional requirements in response to fever, active inflammation, or infection
- Drug side effects.

Consequences of malnutrition are:
- Poor wound and fistula healing
- Increased surgical morbidity and mortality
- Growth retardation in children.

■ Enteral and Parenteral Nutritional Support

Total parenteral nutrition (TPN) and bowel rest have been used to induce remission in some Crohn's disease patients, but this approach deprives the bowel of necessary nutritional substrates and should be reserved for individuals who cannot tolerate enteral nutrition.

Elemental, or monomeric, feedings containing predigested amino acids show short-term effectiveness in management of active Crohn's disease similar to that of corticosteroids, but unpalatability results in attrition of a substantial number of patients on such a regimen.

Other enteral supplements, either oligomeric or polymeric, are better tolerated than monomeric formulas but are less effective than steroids in achieving remission in Crohn's disease. Polymeric enteral supplements can be taken orally or delivered through tubes placed percutaneously into the stomach or the jejunum.

Indications for Total Parenteral Nutrition in Inflammatory Bowel Disease

Patients found to be significantly or severely malnourished who cannot reverse this trend by eating or with enteral supplements either because of intolerance, partial bowel obstruction, nausea, vomiting, or generalized weakness may benefit from TPN. Malnutrition can be documented by subnormal or falling serum levels of albumin, transferrin, or prealbumin or by significant weight loss. Some patients with Crohn's disease cannot tolerate eating or enteral supplementation during a flare of disease and may improve with bowel rest and TPN as primary therapy.

Some patients with Crohn's disease who have undergone extensive small-bowel resection develop "short-bowel syndrome" and may not be able to adequately absorb nutrients taken orally. TPN may be required for a protracted period of time, though the bowel may eventually adapt to the postoperative state and an oral diet.

"End-jejunostomy syndrome," a variant of the short-bowel syndrome, occurs when extensive segments of absorptive small- and large-bowel surfaces have been resected, causing severe fluid and electrolyte deficiencies (particularly magnesium). TPN is often required to replenish fluid and electrolytes, even if nutrients can be absorbed fairly well.

Multiple strictures not amenable to surgical resection may cause pain or vomiting. Long-term TPN may be required. Acute or postoperative fistulas may close more rapidly with bowel rest and a short course of TPN. TPN may also be used for growth retardation in children and adolescents.

Complications of TPN are shown in **Table 9.2**.

TABLE 9.2 — COMPLICATIONS OF TOTAL PARENTERAL NUTRITION
Mechanical
• Catheter embolism
• Hemothorax
• Hydrothorax
• Inadvertent arterial laceration or puncture
• Pneumothorax
• Sepsis
• Venous thrombosis
Metabolic
• Cholestatic liver disease
• Electrolyte disturbances
• Hyperglycemia
• Hypoglycemia (after discontinuing infusion)
• Trace element deficiencies
• Vitamin deficiencies

SUGGESTED READINGS

Greenberger NJ. *Gastrointestinal Disorders: A Pathophysiologic Approach*. Chicago, Ill: Year Book Medical Publishers; 1989:226.

Pastore RL, Wolff BG, Hodge D. Total abdominal colectomy and ileorectal anastomosis for inflammatory bowel disease. *Dis Colon Rectum*. 1997;40:1455-1464.

Podolsky DK. Inflammatory bowel disease. *N Engl J Med*. 2002;347:417-429.

9

10   Ulcerative Colitis

Ulcerative colitis (UC) is a chronic disease that causes inflammation of the colorectal mucosa, typically manifest by relapsing episodes of diarrhea and urgency associated with blood and mucus in the stool. Inflammation is continuous and circumferential, virtually always involving the rectum, and extending a variable distance proximally as far as the cecum. UC is typically divided into three categories based on the extent of the colon that is affected:

- Limited to the rectum or rectosigmoid
- Left-sided colitis, continuing no more proximally than the splenic flexure
- Universal colitis, or pancolitis, involving a larger portion of the colon and often affecting the entire colon.

UC tends to first be identified in a bimodal age distribution. Most patients are diagnosed when they are between 15 and 30 years of age, then a second peak of incidence appears between 55 and 65 years of age.

Epidemiology

Areas of highest incidence of UC include the United Kingdom, the United States, northern Europe and Australia, with Asia, Japan, and South America having the fewest cases. The prevalence did not change significantly from the 1950s through the 1980s, and currently is 2 to 6/100,000 in the United States. Women are slightly more likely to be affected than men, and Jews (especially Ashkenazi Jews) are more prone to develop UC than are non-Jews.

Genetics

Approximately 10% to 20% of patients with UC will have at least one other family member who is affected. Most of the family associations are among first-degree relatives. Affected family members may have either UC or Crohn's disease, although the majority will have UC. Children tend to develop the disease at an earlier age than the affected parent, but siblings usually are diagnosed at similar ages. There tends to be a high concordance rate for the extent of disease and the occurrence or absence of extraintestinal manifestations among close relatives. Concordance rates among monozygotic twins are much lower for UC (6%) than for Crohn's disease (58%), though affected individuals often have a close relative with inflammatory bowel disease.

Etiology

The etiology of UC remains unknown. Infection, food allergy, environmental factors, immune responses to bacterial or autoantigens, and psychosomaticity have been theorized but never proven in studies. Although smoking seems to be protective in patients with UC and UC is less common in smokers than in nonsmokers, an explanation for this relationship has not yet been reached.

Pathology

■ **Macroscopic Features**
  The distribution of colitis is as follows:
  • 20% will have universal colitis, involving the entire colorectum
  • 30% to 40% will have disease limited to the left colon

- 40% to 50% will have only rectal or rectosigmoid colitis
- Occasionally, the cecum will be involved in disease that is otherwise limited to the left colon
- The appendix may occasionally be affected in isolation.

The gross appearance of the mucosa tends to be erythematous, edematous, and granular. With more severe disease, the mucosa becomes intensely hemorrhagic and small ulcers become visible. They may become deeper and irregular with progression of the disease (**Figures 10.1 and 10.2**).

In chronic UC, inflammatory polyps (pseudopolyps) may be identified as a result of regeneration of relatively normal epithelium in the midst of ulcerative disease. Pseudopolyps occur less often in the rectum than more proximally in the colon. When the mucosa is in remission, it may appear normal (**Figure 10.3**), but more often it will look atrophic and featureless, lacking characteristic mucosal folds. There are chronic effects on the muscular layers of the wall resulting in shortening and narrowing of the colonic lumen. Fibrosis and benign strictures are relatively uncommon.

When UC is complicated by toxic megacolon, the colonic wall becomes exceedingly thin and the mucosa is markedly ulcerated, with little intact mucosa remaining. There is a great risk of perforation. Inflammation and vascular congestion may extend into the submucosa. In cases of megacolon with colonic dilatation, ulceration may extend more deeply into the muscularis propria, possibly resulting in ischemic necrosis.

During clinical remission, these histologic abnormalities may reverse almost entirely; however, distorted crypt architecture (**Figures 10.4 and 10.5**) or dropout of glands will typically persist. Fibromuscu-

10

FIGURE 10.1 — SURGICAL FEATURES OF ACTIVE ULCERATIVE COLITIS

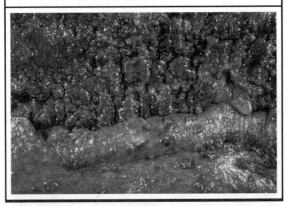

FIGURE 10.2 — COLONOSCOPIC APPEARANCE DURING AN ULCERATIVE COLITIS FLARE

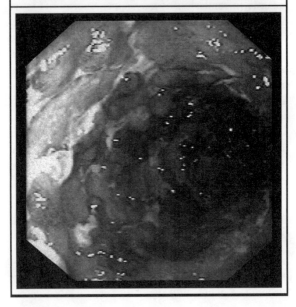

FIGURE 10.3 — NORMAL COLONIC MUCOSA

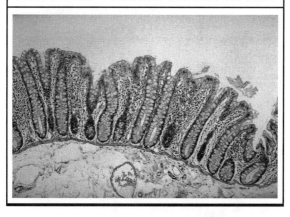

FIGURE 10.4 — MUCOSAL CRYPT DISTORTION IN ULCERATIVE COLITIS

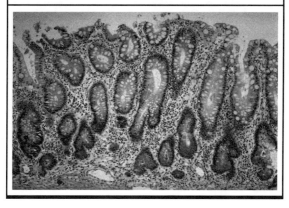

10

FIGURE 10.5 — PRESERVATION OF NORMAL CRYPT ARCHITECTURE IN ACUTE SELF-LIMITED COLITIS

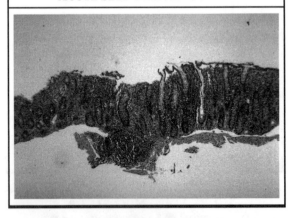

lar hyperplasia of the muscularis mucosae can also be seen in chronic UC.

Symptoms

Persistent bloody diarrhea is the most common symptom of UC, often associated with rectal urgency or tenesmus. Symptoms are indistinguishable from those of infectious diarrhea apart from chronicity in UC.

Aggravating factors include:
- Pregnancy
- Menstruation
- Extremely stressful life events
- Recent discontinuation of smoking.

Physical Findings

In mild-to-moderate disease, physical findings are usually minimal or absent:
- Patients typically appear well with few abnormal findings

- Signs of malnutrition, anemia or other evidence of chronic disease are typically absent, even in moderately severe colitis
- Rectal examination is often normal except that there may be blood recovered.

During severe attacks, findings may include:
- Tachycardia
- Tenderness to palpation over the colon
- Patients whose condition is more severe may appear quite ill, with weight loss and dehydration
- Fever and pallor may occur in severe attacks
- Edema can be seen as a result of hypoproteinemia
- In severe chronic illness, there may be oral thrush, aphthous ulceration, and clubbing of the digits
- Bowel sounds may be reduced and the abdomen may be distended and tympanic
- Perianal disease is far less common than it is in Crohn's disease.

Diagnosis

10

Diagnoses from which UC must be distinguished are shown in **Table 10.1** Stool should be examined for white blood cells (WBCs) and bacteria; additionally, three stool samples should be examined for ova and parasites. The stool should be tested for *Clostridium difficile* infection if the patient has had recent antibiotic exposure or a recent hospitalization. Serologic studies may need to be performed to rule out amebiasis.

Perinuclear-staining antineutrophil cytoplasmic antibodies (pANCA) are present in the serum of nearly 70% of UC patients, while anti-*Saccharomyces cerevisiae* antibodies (ASCA) are rarely found. These antibodies are generally only sought if a specific diagnosis is otherwise elusive or when a pathologic diagnosis of "indefinite colitis" is reached. The presence of pANCA

TABLE 10.1 — DIFFERENTIAL DIAGNOSIS OF ULCERATIVE COLITIS

- Crohn's disease
- Acute self-limited (infectious) colitis:
  - *Salmonella* species
  - *Shigella* species
  - *Campylobacter jejuni*
  - *Yersinia enterocolitica*
  - *Escherichia coli*
- Other infectious colitides:
  - Tuberculous colitis
  - *Clostridium difficile*
  - *Aeromonas* species
  - Amebiasis
  - Schistosomiasis
  - Syphilis
  - *Chlamydia trachomatis*
  - Herpes colitis
  - Cytomegalovirus
- Ischemic colitis
- Radiation colitis
- Collagenous colitis
- Microscopic (lymphocytic) colitis
- Solitary rectal ulcer syndrome (usually associated with rectal prolapse)
- Drug-induced colitis:
  - Nonsteroidal anti-inflammatory drugs (NSAIDs)
  - Gold
  - Penicillamine
  - Salicylates (in which case treating presumed ulcerative colitis [UC] with 5-aminosalicylate compound will make the colitis worse instead of better)
- Other conditions that may clinically mimic UC:
  - Irritable bowel syndrome (IBS)
  - Colon cancer
  - Colon polyps
  - Diverticular disease
  - Factitious diarrhea due to unreported laxative abuse

- Histologic findings that support a diagnosis of UC rather than an acute self-limited colitis (**Figures 10.3, 10.4, and 10.5**):
  - Distorted crypt architecture
  - Crypt atrophy
  - Increased spacing between crypts, with irregularity of the mucosal surface
  - Basal lymphoid aggregates
  - Chronic inflammatory cellular infiltrate

is unrelated to the activity of the colitis and typically remains detectable even after proctocolectomy.

If UC is diagnosed and involves the entire mucosal segment examined at sigmoidoscopy, colonoscopy should be done at a future time to determine the extent of colitis. An endoscopic picture of active UC is shown in **Figure 10.2**. Typical endoscopic findings include:

- Mucosal edema
- Granularity
- Friability
- Erosion or ulceration, with or without inflammatory pseudopolyps
- Continuous involvement of the rectum and extending proximally to a variable extent.

■ Endoscopic Grading Scale

The endoscopic severity of disease can be graded as follows:

- Grade 0 – Normal mucosa
- Grade 1 – Loss of vascular pattern (due to edema)
- Grade 2 – Granular nonfriable mucosa
- Grade 3 – Friability on rubbing
- Grade 4 – Spontaneous bleeding and ulceration.

■ Typical Radiologic Findings

Plain x-rays of the abdomen should be ordered during a severe attack of UC. Thickening of the bowel wall, colonic dilatation, or small-bowel distention may be seen. Proximal retention of stool is common in patients with left-sided disease.

A barium enema is best avoided in a severe attack because of the risk of perforation or of worsening the colitis, particularly if there is colonic dilatation. In mild or moderate illness, however, a double-contrast barium enema is safe and may be valuable in reaching a diagnosis.

An early finding includes fine mucosal granularity with ulceration extending through the mucosa. More chronic disease classically shows a featureless tubular colon with loss of haustration throughout the colon (**Figure 10.6**). The colon may also appear to be short and more narrow than normal.

Polyps in the colon at a barium enema may either be postinflammatory, pseudopolyps, adenomatous polyps, or cancer. A cobblestone pattern can be seen with severe active inflammation.

Laboratory Data

Iron deficiency may occur as a result of chronic blood loss; thus serum iron and total iron-binding capacity should be measured periodically. A severe attack may result in hypokalemia, hypoalbuminemia, and a rise in γ-2-globulin. Abnormal liver function studies may be due to hepatic steatosis (fatty liver), bacteremia, or poor nutrition. Liver studies in a small minority of patients with UC will be persistently abnormal, and many such individuals will eventually be found to have primary sclerosing cholangitis (PSC) (see below).

FIGURE 10.6 — BARIUM ENEMA IN A PATIENT WITH CHRONIC ULCERATIVE COLITIS

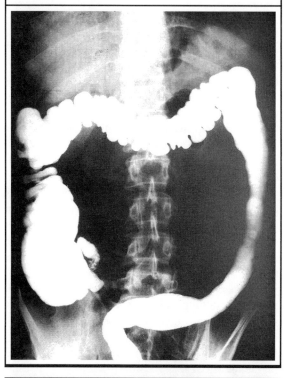

Extraintestinal Manifestations of Ulcerative Colitis

Erythema nodosum is a cutaneous complication that may occur in untreated UC or as a side effect of the sulfapyridine component of sulfasalazine. It appears as multiple tender and inflamed nodules, most often on the anterior surface of the lower legs. Pyoderma gangrenosum occurs in 1% to 2% of UC patients. Skin lesions may occur on either the torso or the extremities as pustules, which may break down, ulcerate, and result in serious necrosis. This problem tends to wax and wane in parallel with activity of the colitis.

Oral aphthous ulcers (found in at least 10% of patients with active colitis) tend to resolve with disease remission. Episcleritis or anterior uveitis occurs in 5% to 8% of patients with active colitis and may require local steroid eye drops to control pain.

Acute arthropathy, seen in 10% to 15% of patients with acute UC, affects larger joints and usually resolves with improvement in colitis. Sacroiliitis, seen in 12% to 15% of patients, may be associated with the HLA-B27 haplotype and may be either asymptomatic or may cause low-back pain.

Ankylosing spondylitis (AS) occurs in 1% to 2% of UC patients. More than 80% of AS patients have the HLA-B27 haplotype. This may cause low-back pain that can be severe and require management with nonsteroidal anti-inflammatory agents, along with physical therapy. It is often associated with uveitis.

Primary sclerosing cholangitis occurs in 3% of UC patients, resulting in cholestatic liver disease, with or without jaundice. It can be diagnosed by liver biopsy, endoscopic retrograde cholangiopancreatography (ERCP), or magnetic resonance cholangiopancreatography (MRCP).

Both intrahepatic and extrahepatic bile ducts may be diseased, causing multiple strictures and areas of dilatation between the strictures anywhere in the biliary tree (**Figure 10.7**). Liver biopsy may demonstrate concentric fibrosis around the bile ductules and, eventually, obliteration of the ducts. Findings that appear similar to those of chronic active hepatitis may be present (with piecemeal necrosis), and chronic inflammatory cells such as lymphocytes and plasma cells may infiltrate the portal tracts. The variant of pericholangitis may simply be the intrahepatic extension of PSC.

**FIGURE 10.7 — ERCP OF A PATIENT
WITH PRIMARY SCLEROSING CHOLANGITIS**

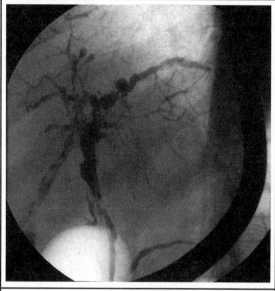

Abbreviations: ERCP, endoscopic retrograde cholangio-pancreatography.

A dominant extrahepatic stricture of the common bile duct and multiple intrahepatic strictures are demonstrated in this radiograph.

Cirrhosis may develop over a period of years after PSC has been diagnosed and may obscure the typical bile duct findings. Seventy percent of patients with PSC have the HLA-DR3-B8 haplotype. Most patients with PSC have extensive colitis, but the course of cholangitis does not parallel that of the colitis. In fact, patients may be diagnosed with PSC many years before UC is diagnosed or not until after total proctocolectomy. The liver disease of PSC eventually becomes progressive, resulting in portal hypertension, fibrosis, and cirrhosis. Cholangiocarcinoma may occur as a complication of PSC and, in fact, 50% of all cases of cholangiocarcinoma are associated with UC.

There is no established, truly effective treatment of PSC. Ursodeoxycholic acid (Actigall) may slow the rate of disease progression. Studies using methotrexate have had equivocal results to date but may be beneficial in some patients. Methotrexate can be taken tid one day each week, at a dose of 0.25 mg/kg/wk. A minority of patients with active inflammatory changes may benefit from steroid therapy. Patients with steatorrhea should be given fat-soluble vitamins (A, D, E, and K) periodically.

Stenting of dominant extrahepatic strictures during ERCP may help to improve the degree of hyperbilirubinemia, and sequential courses of antibiotics (such as erythromycin, trimethoprim/sulfamethoxazole, and ciprofloxacin) may be useful for cholangitis due to intrahepatic strictures. End-stage liver disease can be managed successfully with liver transplantation if cholangiocarcinoma has been excluded.

Management

A management algorithm for UC, developed by the American College of Gastroenterology, is shown in **Figure 10.8**.

■ **Medications**
Oral Aminosalicylates (**Table 10.2**)
Sulfasalazine (*Azulfidine EN*)

In the chemical structure of sulfasalazine (**Figure 10.9**), the 5-aminosalicylic acid (5-ASA) moiety is covalently bound to sulfapyridine. Sulfapyridine is inert but allows 5-ASA to remain in the intestinal lumen until the distal small bowel or the colon, where it is topically effective as an anti-inflammatory agent.

5-ASA alone would be absorbed in the duodenum or proximal jejunum. The covalent bond of 5-ASA to sulfapyridine is cleaved by colonic bacterial azoreductases, releasing the active 5-ASA moiety in the ileum or colon.

Sulfasalazine is far less expensive than newer aminosalicylates, but the likelihood of intolerance due to side effects is much greater with sulfasalazine. Sulfapyridine is the portion of the medication responsible for the majority of side effects. Dose-dependent side effects include:

- Nausea and vomiting
- Anorexia
- Folate malabsorption
- Headache
- Alopecia.

Non–dosage-related side effects include:

- Hypersensitivity rashes (eg, Stevens-Johnson syndrome)
- Hemolytic anemia
- Agranulocytosis
- Hepatotoxicity
- Pancreatitis
- Fibrosing alveolitis
- Male infertility (abnormal sperm morphology and motility, oligospermia)
- Megaloblastic anemia
- Connective tissue disease
- Interstitial nephritis
- Nephrotoxicity.

Sulfasalazine should be administered at a dosage of 3 to 6 g/day divided bid, tid, or qid.

Newer non–sulfa-containing aminosalicylates are devoid of the sulfapyridine fragment and are tolerated by 80% to 90% of patients who cannot tolerate sulfasalazine. The 5-ASA is bound to an inert sub-

FIGURE 10.8 — MEDICAL MANAGEMENT OF ULCERATIVE COLITIS

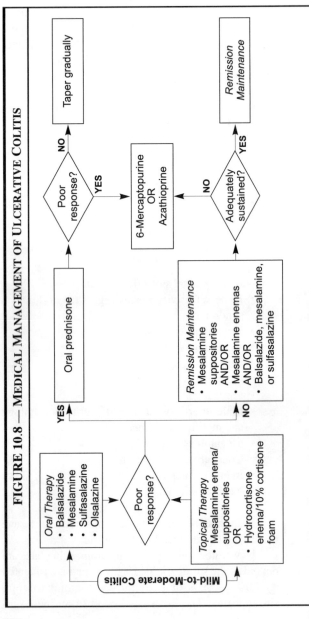

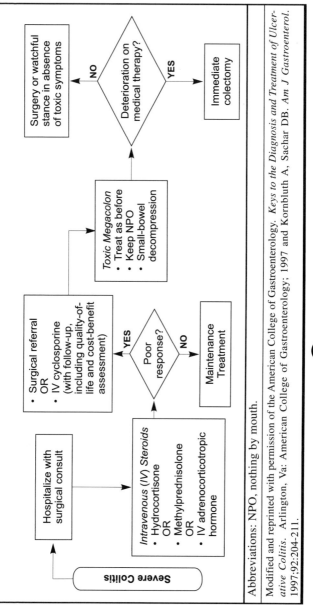

Severe Colitis

Hospitalize with surgical consult

Intravenous (IV) Steroids
- Hydrocortisone OR
- Methylprednisolone OR
- IV adrenocorticotropic hormone

Poor response?

YES →
- Surgical referral OR
- IV cyclosporine (with follow-up, including quality-of-life and cost-benefit assessment)

NO → Maintenance Treatment

Toxic Megacolon
- Treat as before
- Keep NPO
- Small-bowel decompression

Deterioration on medical therapy?

NO → Surgery or watchful stance in absence of toxic symptoms

YES → Immediate colectomy

Abbreviations: NPO, nothing by mouth.

Modified and reprinted with permission of the American College of Gastroenterology. *Keys to the Diagnosis and Treatment of Ulcerative Colitis.* Arlington, Va: American College of Gastroenterology; 1997 and Kornbluth A, Sachar DB. *Am J Gastroenterol.* 1997;92:204-211.

10

147

TABLE 10.2 — ORAL 5-AMINOSALICYLATE DRUGS

Generic/*Trade* Name	Chemical Composition	Area(s) of Release in the GI Tract	Formulation
Sulfasalazine/*Azulfidine*	Sulfapyridine and 5-ASA	Colon	Tablet
Olsalazine/*Dipentum*	5-ASA dimer	Distal ileum, colon	Gelatin capsule
Balsalazide/*Colazal*	5-ASA + 4-aminobenzoyl-glycine + β-alanine	Colon, particularly the distal colon	Capsule
Mesalamine			
Asacol	5-ASA	Distal ileum, colon	Eudragit polymer-coated tablet, dissolves at neutral pH
Pentasa	5-ASA	Duodenum, jejunum, ileum, and colon	Ethylcellulose-coated beads (microgranules) in a capsule
Rowasa	5-ASA	Rectum (suppository) or distal colon (enema)	Enema, suppository

Abbreviations: GI, gastrointestinal; 5-ASA, 5-aminosalicylate.

Adapted from: Stotland BR, et al. *Hosp Pract.* 1998;33:141-144, 149-151, 156.

stance or to another molecule of 5-ASA, instead of to a sulfa moiety (**Figure 10.9**). The decision of which to prescribe is probably best made based on the extent of disease, considering the differences in their mechanisms of release of the active moiety.

Olsalazine (Dipentum)

Olsalazine is a dimer of 5-ASA. It should be administered at a dosage of 250 to 500 mg po bid. Its effectiveness is limited by the side effect of diarrhea; this may be preventable by building up to the goal dosage over several days.

Balsalazide (Colazal)

Balsalazide, recently approved for use in the United States, is 5-ASA bound to inert carrier 4-aminobenzoyl-b-alanine (4-ABA) by a diazo bond that is cleaved by colonic bacterial azoreductase. The usual dosage is 6.75 g/day (three 750-mg capsules po tid), providing 2.4 g mesalamine daily.

Virtually all of the 5-ASA in balsalazide is released in the colon, making it useful in UC of any extent. Based on initial clinical studies, release of 5-ASA is greater in the colon than with pH-dependent mechanisms that begin to release it more proximally. Symptom relief may be more rapid with balsalazide than with the other forms of mesalamine and side effects appear to be less common. These factors may allow balsalazide to be used in place of mesalamine enemas or suppositories for left-sided colitis, which may improve patient compliance.

Mesalamine

Asacol is 5-ASA encapsulated in a pH-sensitive matrix, which prevents release of the active drug until the terminal ileum is reached. The usual dosage for the

FIGURE 10.9 — CHEMICAL STRUCTURE OF THE AMINOSALICYLATES

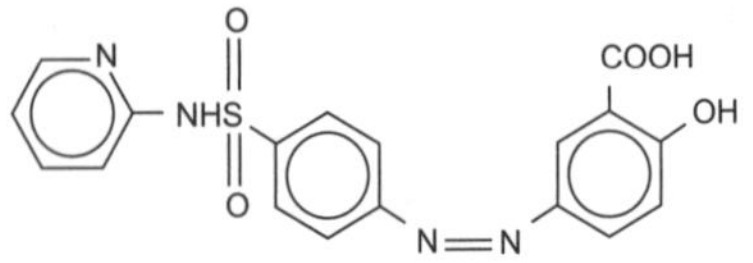

Sulfasalazine (Azulfidine)

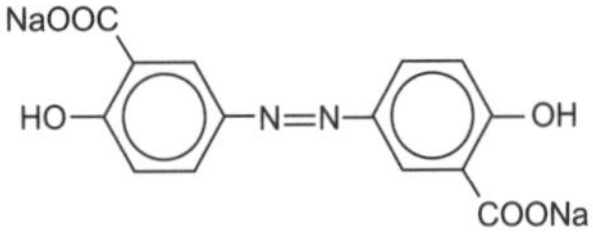

Dimer of 5-ASA
Olsalazine (Dipentum)

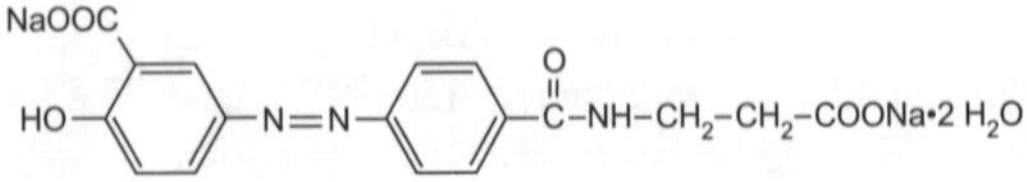

5-ASA + 4-aminobenzoyl–β-alanine
Balsalazide (Colazal)

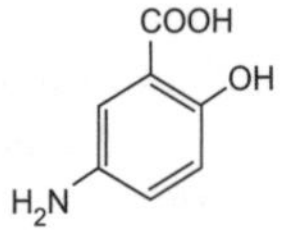

5-ASA
Mesalamine (Asacol, Pentasa, and Rowasa)

Abbreviations: 5-ASA, 5-aminosalicylic acid.

treatment of mild to moderately active disease is 2.4 g/day (two 400-mg capsules po tid), while the usual dosage for the maintenance of remission is 1.6 g/day. Although higher doses may be required in some instances, an attempt at tapering to the minimum effective dose is most appropriate. This formulation delivers 5-ASA throughout the colon and is effective in pancolitis.

Pentasa capsules disintegrate in the stomach to form hundreds of ethylcellulose-coated granules that are released throughout the gastrointestinal tract. This is the best formulation of 5-ASA for treatment of inflammation in the proximal small bowel since more medication is released in the small bowel than with other 5-ASA formulations. The dosage is 4 g/day (four 250-mg capsules po qid).

Topical Aminosalicylate Therapy

Suppositories, foams, and enemas may be used to deliver topical aminosalicylate therapy. Advantages of topical therapy include:

- A more rapid response time
- A less-frequent dosing schedule
- Delivery of medication to the affected area only, resulting in fewer systemic side effects. Suppositories deliver medication a distance of 10 to 15 cm, foam 15 to 20 cm, and enemas often reach the splenic flexure.

Disadvantages of topical aminosalicylate therapy include:

- Greater expense than oral therapy
- Less desirable means of taking medication.

Mesalamine enemas (Rowasa), 4 g nightly, deliver medication directly to the rectum and as far proximal as the splenic flexure in more than 90% of patients (effective in inducing and maintaining remission in proctitis and left-sided colitis). Systemic side effects are rare. Although it is usually effective within 3 to 21 days, treatment should be continued for at least 3 to 6 weeks. Some patients will require longer-term therapy (up to 6 months) to achieve remission. Relapses are common in UC after discontinuing therapy; changing administration to every other night or every third night may help to reduce the likelihood of relapse or delay it. Mesalamine suppositories (Canasa) should be used at a dosage of 500 mg rectally bid and are effective in treating proctitis and maintaining remission. Patients can be advised to use the suppositories after a bowel movement early in the day and at bedtime, if possible. These topical agents may also be useful in combination with oral mesalamine or balsalazide in UC for more extensive colitis.

Corticosteroids

Corticosteroids impede the inflammatory response by blocking production of arachidonic acid from phospholipids. Prednisone, administered at 40 to 60 mg daily (or an equivalent dosage of methylprednisolone, hydrocortisone, or dexamethasone) can induce remission in 70% to 80% of acute flares of inflammatory bowel disease (IBD) in which aminosalicylate therapy has failed.

Some of the side effects of corticosteroids are:
- Adrenal suppression
- Osteoporosis
- Glucose intolerance
- Osteonecrosis
- Cataracts.

While these side effects may be acceptable in an acutely ill patient or in one who has failed to respond to aminosalicylates, they far outweigh the benefit in maintenance therapy.

Means of reducing side effects of systemic corticosteroids include:
- Rapid tapering of dosage
- Alternate-day administration
- Topical application (suppositories, foam, enemas)
- Use of rapidly metabolized first-pass steroids (eg, budesonide, tixocortol pivalate, fluticasone

propionate) which can reduce or, in the case of fluticasone, eliminate suppression of the corticoadrenal axis

- Bone destruction may possibly be reduced with concurrent use of calcium (at least 1000 mg/day) and vitamin D 400 IU (available in a typical multivitamin). Bisphosphonates, including alendronate sodium (Fosamax), can also be used for this purpose.

The systemic side effects of topical corticosteroids are no worse than those of placebo. Retention enemas and foams are available with hydrocortisone (eg, Cortenema, Cortifoam, Proctofoam-HC) and prednisolone. A hydrocortisone enema (Cortenema), 100 mg, or a 10% cortisone foam (Cortifoam) is effective in treating distal colitis, but neither has been approved for maintenance of remission.

Antibiotics

Metronidazole interferes directly with the inflammatory process in addition to its antibacterial properties. It is effective in the treatment of pouchitis, which may occur after total proctocolectomy and creation of an ileal reservoir. It is also effective in the treatment of *C difficile* infection, which may occasionally be responsible for a flare-up of IBD. In general, however, it is ineffective in treating active UC.

Immunomodulators

Azathioprine

Azathioprine (Imuran) and its active metabolite 6-mercaptopurine (6-MP) (Purinethol) are similar in their mechanism of activity, efficacy, and toxicity profile. They function by inhibiting purine metabolism and may interfere with nucleic acid metabolism in cell-mediated inflammatory responses to antigenic stimuli.

One of these agents should be considered when steroids cannot be tapered or discontinued, and they are especially effective in controlling distal UC in an effort to delay surgical resection. Utility is lessened by a slow onset of action; it requires at least 3 months of therapy for effectiveness to be seen and often takes as long as 6 months. However, a recent preliminary study showed intravenous (IV) azathioprine at dosages of 1200 mg over 36 hours, followed by an oral dosage of 500 to 100 mg/day to induce remission in as little as 4 weeks. Dosage for azathioprine is 50 mg/day or up to a maximum of 2 mg/kg/day. The 6-MP dosage is 50 mg/day or 1.5 mg/kg/day. Leukopenia is used by some practitioners to determine the maximal tolerated dose.

Side effects include:

- Bone marrow toxicity (2%)—dose-dependent effect and may be lethal; requires periodic monitoring of blood counts while on therapy. One possible monitoring scheme would be to check complete blood count with differential weekly for 4 to 6 weeks, then if WBCs remain ≥4,000, the interval can be increased gradually to once every 3 months
- Allergic reactions (2%)
- Pancreatitis (3% to 5%)
- Infections (2%)
- Hepatitis (rare)
- Apparent increase in spontaneous miscarriages and possible increased risk of birth defects when a mother takes 6-MP during pregnancy or if the father takes it within 3 months of partner's pregnancy.

Azathioprine or 6-MP can also be used in UC for maintenance of remission in nonsurgical candidates. Fear of delayed occurrence of malignancies with the use of these agents does not appear to be justified based on long-term studies. Patients taking these medications are, however, at risk of opportunistic infections, as is the case with other immunosuppressive drugs.

The immunosuppressive characteristics of 6-MP are due to its metabolite 6-thioguanine (6-TG), produced via a chemical reaction that is suppressed by the enzyme thiopurine methyltranferase (TPMT) (**Figure 10.10**). A 6-TG level of at least 230 pmol has been associated with improved response in several studies. Homozygous TPMT deficiency, which occurs in one in 300 individuals, may result in prohibitively excessive 6-TG levels (>400 pmol), resulting in leukopenia. Such individuals cannot receive 6-MP. Heterozygotes for TPMT deficiency typically can be treated with very low doses of 6-MP. Those with increased activity of TPMT cause 6-MP to be converted to 6-methyl mercaptopurine (6MMP) rather than 6-TG, resulting in subtherapeutic levels of 6-TG and the potential for 6MMP-induced hepatotoxicity.

Cyclosporine A

This medication selectively suppresses cellular immunity by inhibiting interleukin-2. Its onset of action of 1 to 2 weeks is more rapid than that of azathioprine or 6-MP.

In UC, cyclosporine A is often effective in achieving remission in poor surgical candidates who have failed to respond to other aggressive medical management, including a week of IV corticosteroids. Remission is achieved in over 80% of patients with severe UC within 1 week, and remission is maintained in over half of such patients. However, 70% of patients will still require colectomy within 1 to 2 years. The best role of this medication is probably as a temporary measure until either colectomy can be performed or immunomodulatory medication (azathioprine, 6-MP) becomes effective.

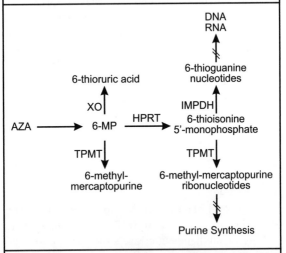
Side effects of cyclosporine A include:

- Hypertension
- Seizures (especially in patients with hypocholesterolemia)
- Infections (may be serious or even fatal)
- Paresthesias
- Tremor
- Cholestasis
- Anorexia
- Vomiting
- Nausea

- Gingival hyperplasia
- Hypertrichosis
- Renal damage with decreased glomerular filtration rate
- Hypomagnesemia, hyperkalemia (may be irreversible in some cases).

Methotrexate

Methotrexate is a folic acid antagonist that has both anti-inflammatory and antimetabolite activity. It is moderately effective in UC, studied at a dosage of 25 mg IM weekly x 12 weeks, then 25 mg po weekly. A better early response rate is observed in Crohn's disease than in UC, however. Most responders do so within 8 to 10 weeks of initiating therapy. Methotrexate is useful as a steroid-sparing agent in some patients.

Omega-3 Fatty Acids

This group includes eicosapentaenoic acid and other substances derived from fish oils. They serve as anti-inflammatory agents through chemical similarity to arachidonic acid. These agents may be effective in the management of active UC but not in the maintenance of remission.

■ Management Based on Clinical Severity

Decisions are based on the clinical severity of disease and on the extent of colitis. The clinical severity of colitis is determined as follows:

- Mild disease: less than four stools daily, with or without blood, with no systemic signs of toxicity and a normal erythrocyte sedimentation rate (ESR)
- Moderate disease: more than four stools a day; minimal signs of toxicity

- Severe disease: more than six stools per day; evidence of toxicity, including fever, tachycardia, anemia, or an elevated ESR.

Mild-to-Moderate Distal Colitis
Oral Aminosalicylates

Oral aminosalicylates are effective in up to 80% of patients, usually within 2 to 4 weeks. Sulfasalazine (Azulfidine) or non–sulfa-containing aminosalicylates can be used, including:
- Balsalazide (Colazal), 2.25 g po tid
- Mesalamine (Asacol), 800 mg po tid
- Mesalamine (Pentasa), 1 g po qid
- Olsalazine (Dipentum), 250 to 500 mg po bid, though efficacy has not been thoroughly evaluated because of the side effect of diarrhea.

Topical Therapy

Topical therapy includes:
- Topical mesalamine (Canasa 500-mg suppository bid) is effective in treating proctitis and maintaining remission. Rowasa enemas, 1 to 4 g nightly, can induce and maintain remission in distal colitis
- Topical corticosteroids (100-mg hydrocortisone enema [Cortenema], or as a 10% cortisone foam [Cortifoam]); effective in treating distal colitis, but not proven in maintenance of remission.

Oral Corticosteroid Therapy

Failures after above therapy may necessitate use of oral prednisone up to 60 mg/day, or its equivalent.

Maintenance of Remission

For maintenance of remission in distal colitis, the following options are available:

- Mesalamine suppositories 500 mg pr bid
- Mesalamine enemas 4 g pr hs
- Sulfasalazine 2 to 4 g po daily (divided bid to qid)
- Balsalazide (Colazal) 2.25 g po tid
- Mesalamine (Pentasa) 1 g po qid
- Mesalamine (Asacol) 800 mg po bid.

Topical corticosteroids have not proven effective for maintenance of remission.

Mild-to-Moderate Universal Colitis:
Active Disease

Oral therapy is required, possibly in combination with topical therapy, and effectiveness is dose-related:

- Sulfasalazine 4 to 6 g/day is effective within 4 weeks in about 80% of patients
- Other oral aminosalicylates are equally effective (Asacol, Colazal, Dipentum, Pentasa)
- Topical therapy added to oral therapy often brings more prompt relief of rectal symptoms
- Oral steroids are necessary in some patients — oral prednisone, 20 to 60 mg/day can be used; one approach is to start with 40 to 60 mg/day until clinical improvement, then decrease daily dose by 5 to 10 mg each week until dose is 20 mg/day, then decrease daily dose by 2.5 mg weekly until discontinuation is possible.
- Azathioprine (Imuran), 1.5 to 2.5 mg/kg/day or 6-MP (Purinethol) is effective in achieving and maintaining remission in patients who do not respond to or cannot be fully weaned off corticosteroids; onset of action is slow, with optimal effect often not seen for 3 to 6 months.

Mild-to-Moderate Universal Colitis:
Maintenance of Remission

All of the aminosalicylates are effective in reducing relapses. Sulfasalazine is most effective at a higher dosage (1 g po qid) if tolerated. Doses of the other aminosalicylates of up to 4.8 g/day of 5-ASA are better tolerated and similarly effective. Permanent maintenance therapy is advised, though attempts to discontinue medication may be reasonable if the first flare is mild. Avoid steroids for chronic use, if at all possible.

Azathioprine or 6-MP can reduce steroid doses in patients who are steroid dependent and can be added to aminosalicylates when they are ineffective alone. These agents can reduce the 12-month relapse rate from 59% (on placebo) to 36%. The benefit of long-term use of immunomodulators must be compared with colectomy, considering potential medication side effects.

Smoking appears to maintain remissions and control flares of UC. It may prevent the need for colectomy in some individuals in whom medical therapy has failed after cessation of smoking.

Severe (Fulminant) Colitis

The patient must be hospitalized if there is a failure to respond adequately to oral corticosteroid (prednisone 40 to 60 mg/day), aminosalicylates (sulfasalazine 4 to 6 g/day or mesalamine at up to 4.8 g/day), or topical therapy alone or in combination. Once in hospital, IV steroids (hydrocortisone 300 mg/day or methylprednisolone 48 mg/day) should be given either continuously or in divided doses.

Adrenocorticotropic hormone (ACTH) can be used in place of steroids if the patient has not received steroids for at least 1 month. The success rate of medical therapy in this setting is about 40%.

Early surgical consultation is appropriate. If the patient has signs of clinical toxicity, such as fever, leukocytosis, progressively worsening symptoms, or toxic megacolon, narcotics and anticholinergic agents should be avoided as they may worsen colonic atony and dilatation. Total parenteral nutrition should *not* be used routinely. Enteral nutrition is effective in delivering necessary short-chain fatty acids to colonic enterocytes. Parenteral nutrition can be used in addition to enteral nutrition in states of significant malnutrition.

An oral aminosalicylate is only of value if the patient was already taking it and is able to tolerate oral intake. There is no proven benefit in adding it *de novo* to steroids in a patient with severe colitis.

Patients who fail to respond to 7 to 10 days of maximal medical therapy are unlikely to respond to a longer similar course. In this situation, options include:

- Surgery (colectomy)
- Investigational therapy, such as IV cyclosporine (4 mg/kg/day), which is effective in 80% of patients who are able to avoid surgery for the acute flare.

Toxic Megacolon

Colonic dilatation is termed "toxic megacolon" when the transverse colonic diameter is larger than 6 cm or cecal diameter is larger than 9 cm in the setting of an acute flare of colitis. Management includes:

- Nothing by mouth (NPO)
- Rectal tube
- Small-bowel decompression tube (if small-bowel ileus is apparent)
- Instructing the patient to rotate between prone (knee-elbow), supine, and lateral positions frequently to facilitate evacuation of flatus
- Broad-spectrum antibiotics to limit complications in the event of perforation.

Indications for surgery for toxic megacolon include:

- Clinical, radiologic or laboratory deterioration while on medical therapy
- Failure to demonstrate improvement within 72 hours (controversial).

Indications for Surgery in Ulcerative Colitis

Absolute indications for surgery in UC include:
- Exsanguinating hemorrhage (due to diffuse ulceration):
  - Total proctocolectomy, if condition permits
  - Subtotal colectomy if restorative ileorectostomy is planned (though 12% of such patients will bleed from the remaining rectal segment)
- Perforation (occurs in 2% to 3% of hospitalized UC patients in tertiary referral centers):
  - The most highly lethal complication of toxic colonic dilatation (or may occur in the absence of dilatation)
  - Operation of choice in this setting is subtotal colectomy with a rectosigmoid mucous fistula or Hartmann's pouch
- Documented or strongly suspected cancer (**Table 10.3**):
  - High-grade dysplasia (HGD) or low-grade dysplasia (LGD) in flat mucosa dysplasia associated with a lesion or mass (DALM) is a clear indication for colectomy
  - Even LGD in flat mucosa has a great enough eventual risk of malignancy that it should be considered an indication for colectomy (19% incidence of cancer in colectomy specimens after surgery done for LGD, and 5-year predictive value for eventual progression to HGD or cancer is as high as 54%)
  - Stricture not passable with a colonoscope is associated with carcinoma 25% of the time

and should be evaluated surgically if cancer cannot be excluded otherwise

- Severe (fulminant) colitis or toxic megacolon that fails to respond to maximal IV medical therapy
- Less severe but medically intractable symptoms that result in physical debility or psychosocial dysfunction
- Intolerable medication side effects (especially with steroids), although a majority of these patients will respond to immunosuppressive drugs such as 6-MP or azathioprine
- Severe progressive pyoderma gangrenosum (when skin disease parallels the colitis) or hemolytic anemia refractory to steroids and splenectomy.

Surgical Options

Any colonic surgery required in a patient with UC involving more than the rectosigmoid should include removal of the entire colon and, if possible, the rectum. Total proctocolectomy and eventual ileoanal anastomosis are the procedures of choice, because they not only remove the entire segment of bowel susceptible to recurrent colitis, but eliminate the risk of colorectal cancer as well (**Figures 10.11 and 10.12**). Older patients or individuals with inadequate anal sphincter function may opt instead for a total proctocolectomy with a permanent ileostomy to avoid the risk of fecal incontinence after ileoanal anastomosis.

Subtotal colectomy (leaving the rectum *in situ*) with a primary ileorectal anastomosis is a one-step procedure that can be done in patients in whom a proctocolectomy and ileoanal anastomosis cannot or should not be done. The remaining rectal mucosa should be screened periodically for colon cancer, and recurrent colitis may occur in this segment.

TABLE 10.3 — CANCER RISK BASED ON DYSPLASIA IN COLONOSCOPIC BIOPSIES IN INFLAMMATORY BOWEL DISEASE

Diagnosis	Probability of Finding Cancer if Colectomy Is Done Immediately (%)	Probability of Finding Cancer if Colectomy Is Done After Follow-up (%)
DALM	43	NA
High-grade dysplasia	42	32
Low-grade dysplasia	19	8
Indefinite for dysplasia	NA	9
No dysplasia	NA	2

Abbreviations: DALM, dysplasia associated with a lesion or mass; NA, not applicable.

Adapted from: Itzkowitz SH. *Gastroenterol Clin North Am.* 1997;26:129-139.

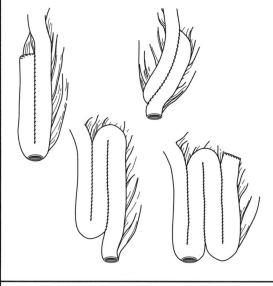

Adapted from: Becker JM, Parodi JE. Total colectomy with preservation of the anal sphincter. *Surg Annu.* 1989;21:263.

Recommendations for Cancer Surveillance

Annual surveillance colonoscopy should be initiated after 8 to 10 years of colitis, extending proximal to the sigmoid colon (whether it is left-sided or universal colitis) with biopsies taken at 10-cm intervals. Screening at 2-year intervals will miss some early cancers and is especially hazardous in long-standing disease. Screening colonoscopy should be avoided during periods of clinical relapse as active inflammation may obscure neoplastic changes.

FIGURE 10.12 — ILEAL "J" POUCH: ANAL ANASTOMOSIS

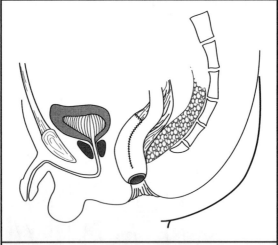

The 2-loop ileal pouch is simple to construct, provides adequate storage capacity, and is evacuated spontaneously and fully.

Patients with only proctitis or proctosigmoiditis are not at increased cancer risk and should be screened as average-risk individuals based on age and other risk factors that may be present.

After 10 years of universal colitis, cancer risk increases by 0.5% to 1% per year. After 30 to 40 years of disease, the cancer risk in left-sided colitis equals that of universal colitis.

Colitis-associated cancers (in comparison with other colorectal cancers):

- Tend to more frequently be multiple, broadly infiltrating, anaplastic, and uniformly distributed throughout the colon
- Occur in flat mucosa, rather than arising in an adenomatous polyp

- Occur in a much younger population than does cancer in the general population.

Premalignant findings in surveillance biopsies may include:
- Definite dysplasia (either low- or high-grade); if confirmed, colectomy is indicated
- Indefinite dysplasia (if considered so after review by an expert pathologist); necessitates more frequent surveillance
- Regenerative atypia due to inflammation and repair; can be mistaken for neoplastic dysplasia.

SUGGESTED READING

American College of Gastroenterology. *Keys to the Diagnosis and Treatment of Ulcerative Colitis*. Arlington, Va: American College of Gastroenterology; 1997.

Jewell DP. Ulcerative colitis. In: Feldman M, Friedman LS, Sleisenger MH, eds. *Sleisenger and Fordtran's Gastrointestinal and Liver Disease*: *Pathophysiology/Diagnosis/Management*. 7th ed. Philadelphia, Pa: WB Saunders Co; 2002:2039-2067.

Kornbluth A, Sachar DB. Ulcerative colitis practice guidelines in adults. American College of Gastroenterology, Practice Parameters Committee. *Am J Gastroenterol*. 1997;92:204-211.

Pemberton JH, Phillips SF. Ileostomy and its alternatives. In: Feldman M, Friedman LS, Sleisenger MH, eds. *Sleisenger and Fordtran's Gastrointestinal and Liver Disease*: *Pathophysiology/Diagnosis/Management*. 7th ed. Philadelphia, Pa: WB Saunders Co; 2002:2068-2079.

Podolsky DK. Inflammatory bowel disease. *N Engl J Med*. 2002;347:417-429. Review.

10

11   Crohn's Disease

Crohn's disease is a chronic transmural inflammatory condition that may affect any part of the digestive tract, from the lips to the anus. The most frequently affected areas are the:

- Ileum
- Colon
- Perianal area.

Common symptoms of this disease include:

- Diarrhea
- Abdominal pain
- Weight loss
- Gastrointestinal (GI) bleeding.

Extraintestinal organs are often affected, especially with Crohn's colitis. Crohn's disease is incurable, even with surgical resection, and tends to be associated with periodic remissions and relapses.

Treatment is primarily pharmacologic, with surgery being reserved for disease that has failed to respond to an adequate trial of medication. Affected areas that have undergone surgery present an even greater risk of recurrent disease, typically just proximal to the anastomosis. Although the disease has historically been referred to as granulomatous colitis, granulomatous enteritis, regional enteritis, or terminal ileitis, these terms have been abandoned because granulomas, pathologic hallmarks of the disease, are not necessarily identifiable in all patients, and the affected areas of the GI tract vary from patient to patient.

Familial associations are much stronger with Crohn's disease than with ulcerative colitis (UC). The relative risk of Crohn's disease developing in siblings of afflicted patients is 17 to 35 times that in the general population. Monozygotic twins have a 58% concordance rate for Crohn's disease, although pure Mendelian inheritance does not appear to describe the genetic link. Like UC, Crohn's disease is much more common in Jews (especially Ashkenazi Jews) than in non-Jews.

The onset of disease is greatest in people in their teens and 20s, and there may be a second peak in the 70s. Smokers have a 2- to 5-fold increased risk of developing the disease. The incidence has increased significantly since the 1950s in the United States and other westernized countries, and currently is 5/100,000 with a prevalence of 50/100,000.

Etiology

The underlying etiology of Crohn's disease remains obscure. Environment and heredity have been implicated over the years but are unproven. Associations with the measles virus and with *Mycobacterium paratuberculosis* are possible. A weak genetic association may exist since relatives of individuals with Crohn's disease have an increased risk of developing either Crohn's disease or UC (with Crohn's being more likely) and first-degree relatives are at greatest risk.

Stressful life events have not conclusively been associated with either the etiology or exacerbation of flares of Crohn's disease.

Pathology

Active Crohn's disease causes injury to intestinal crypts, resulting in cryptitis and crypt abscesses with an acute inflammatory cell infiltrate. The distribution of these crypt lesions tends to be focal, as opposed to UC, in which the entire segment of diseased colon is microscopically, if not endoscopically, affected. Crypt injury evolves into microscopic mucosal ulceration associated with inflammation in deeper levels of the intestinal wall. A chronic inflammatory cell infiltrate (with lymphocytes and plasma cells) may be seen, and crypt architecture becomes distorted with dropout of crypts. Macrophages organize into noncaseating granulomas, which can be found in all layers of the bowel wall from the mucosa to the serosa, as well as in lymph nodes, the mesentery, peritoneum, liver, and peripheral tissues. Granulomas, though considered a hallmark of Crohn's disease, are only present in about half of affected patients (**Figure 11.1**).

FIGURE 11.1 — HISTOLOGIC SLIDE DEMONSTRATING GRANULOMAS AND DISTORTED CRYPT ARCHITECTURE IN CROHN'S DISEASE

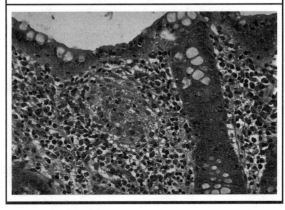

Localized areas of ulceration (aphthous ulcers) may be present on any mucosal surface, including the mouth, and may show granulomas. Extensive deep linear ulcerations and heaped-up edematous tissue in between the ulcerated areas may result in a "cobblestone" appearance of the bowel wall. More advanced disease is associated with thickening of the wall, with fibrosis and often stenosis, described as a "lead pipe" on barium studies (**Figure 11.2**). Stenotic areas may result in bowel obstruction that must be distinguished from malignancy. Stenosis may also be the result of thickening of the mesentery that can eventually scar down and fix individual segments of the bowel. Inflammation of the serosal and mesenteric surfaces causes adhesion of one bowel loop to another. Extension of ulcers through adherent areas into adjacent structures produces fistulas.

Anatomic Distribution

The small bowel is affected in 75% of patients, nearly all of whom have terminal ileal inflammation.

FIGURE 11.2 — BARIUM STUDY SHOWING SMALL-BOWEL CROHN'S DISEASE

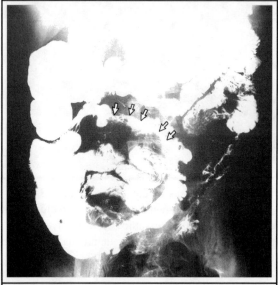

Stricture of Crohn's disease is marked with arrows.

The small bowel is the only area involved in 30% to 40% of patients. Both the small and large bowels are involved in 40% to 50% of patients. Colitis alone is seen in 15% to 25% of patients, and 25% of this group have disease throughout the entire colon. Rectal sparing is common, in contradistinction to UC, in which the rectum is virtually always diseased. Perirectal and perianal disease is present in about 33% of patients, particularly in those who have colitis.

Upper GI (usually gastroduodenal) involvement is rarely present in the absence of disease in the small bowel or colon. Uninvolved "skip" areas in the GI tract distinguish Crohn's disease from UC, in which the entire mucosal surface is histologically abnormal, even if segments appear endoscopically or radiographically unaffected.

Signs and Symptoms

The clinical features of Crohn's disease are described in **Table 11.1**. Terminal ileal disease typically presents with right lower-quadrant abdominal pain and diarrhea, which is usually free of blood. Right lower-quadrant abdominal tenderness, fever, and a palpable mass in a child or young adult may mimic the pain of acute appendicitis. Pain is usually colicky and may be relieved with a bowel movement.

Diarrhea is often, but not always, present. Multiple explanations for the diarrhea are possible:

- Bacterial overgrowth may occur due to stasis of intestinal contents due to partial obstruction.
- Fistulization may allow short-circuiting of intestinal content, bypassing absorptive surfaces in the small bowel.
- Bile-acid diarrhea may be the result of the ileum being unable to absorb bile acids properly, and a diseased colon may not be able to absorb water adequately.

TABLE 11.1 — CLINICAL FEATURES OF CROHN'S DISEASE

Typical History Before Diagnosis
- Chronic diarrhea
- Abdominal pain
- Anorexia
- Weight loss
- Unexplained fever
- Aphthous ulcers of lips and mouth
- Arthralgias (truncal or in extremities)
- Epigastric pain, nausea, vomiting, or gastric outlet obstruction if gastroduodenal involvement
- In children, retarded growth, delayed or failed development of secondary sexual characteristics

Signs
- Pallor
- Cachexia
- Clubbing of the digits
- Abdominal mass or tenderness
- Signs of bowel obstruction
- Perianal fissures, fistulae, or abscesses
- Extraintestinal manifestations:
  - Skin: erythema nodosum and pyoderma gangrenosum
  - Eyes: uveitis (associated with scleroconjunctivitis)
  - Jaundice: may be due to sclerosing cholangitis
- Hypercoagulability
- Metabolic disorders due to malabsorption:
  - Nephrolithiasis (due to hyperoxaluria after small-intestine resection)
  - Cholelithiasis
  - Metabolic bone disease due to vitamin D or calcium malabsorption
  - Anemia due to iron, folate, or vitamin B_{12} malabsorption

Presentation in Childhood
- Gastrointestinal (GI) symptoms similar to those of adults
- Systemic and extraintestinal symptoms may overshadow GI symptoms:
  - Arthritis and arthralgias are very common in children and adolescents and may substantially precede the onset of GI symptoms of Crohn's disease

- Systemic symptoms:
  - Failure to thrive (delayed growth)*
  - Delayed development of secondary sexual characteristics*
  - Fever of unknown origin
  - Unexplained anemia
  - Weight loss
  - Poor oral intake

Effects of Crohn's Disease on Fertility and Pregnancy
- May cause a mild reduction in fertility for a variety of reasons:
  - Dyspareunia due to perineal disease
  - Diminished libido
  - Ovulatory irregularity due to chronic illness or malnutrition
  - Adnexal involvement by adjacent inflammatory disease may rarely cause tubal occlusion
  - In men, sulfasalazine can cause reversible oligospermia and sperm dysmotility
- Pregnancy and Crohn's disease:
  - 12% spontaneous abortion rate
  - 5% will require a therapeutic abortion
  - 2% stillbirth rate
  - No increased rate of congenital abnormalities
  - Vaginal delivery can be potentially problematic if patient has perineal Crohn's disease, but otherwise vaginal delivery can still be attempted
- Effect of pregnancy on Crohn's disease:
  - Most women in remission at time of pregnancy will remain in remission
  - 25% may relapse, usually in first trimester
  - Remission rarely occurs in women who become pregnant with active Crohn's disease despite treatment
- All of the medications used in the management of inflammatory bowel disease can be used during pregnancy if necessary to maintain the mother's health to maximize likelihood of safe pregnancy and delivery

11

* These symptoms can be reversed with effective medical or surgical therapy of the underlying disease, provided that this is done before epiphyseal closures in the teenage years.

- Perianal disease may be associated with urgency and tenesmus due to reduced compliance of the sphincter muscles.

Fever is usually associated with a suppurative complication such as an abscess. Weight loss is frequent and may be substantial. It is usually the result of anorexia, diarrhea, and/or the fear of eating. Malabsorption may be the result of bacterial overgrowth, short-bowel syndrome from extensive small-bowel resection, or extensive small-bowel disease. It may also be an indication of malignancy.

Gross bleeding is far less common than with UC and is usually due to deep ulceration, particularly in the colon.

■ Disease Patterns
Fibrostenotic/Obstructive Disease
The classic radiographic finding of a "string sign" is due to intermittent obstruction from bowel wall edema and spasm that typically causes postprandial pain. This eventually progresses to fibrosis and stenosis, often with stricturing. Stricturing may replace diarrhea with constipation and may further progress to bowel obstruction. In patients with severe disease involving the stomach and duodenum, chronic gastric outlet obstruction may clinically mimic peptic ulcer disease.

Fistulous/Penetrating Disease
Sinus tracts can result from disease extending through the serosa. If the sinus tracts end in a blind area, this results in an abscess, causing:
- Abdominal pain
- Fever
- A tender, palpable mass.

Inflamed serosal surfaces may become adherent and disease may penetrate into other loops of intestine, resulting in a fistula (most often ileoileal, ileocecal, or ileosigmoid).

Fistulas are best diagnosed with barium studies, with lower yields obtained when sought endoscopically. Longer gastrocolic or duodenocolic fistulas are rare, but can be associated with severe malabsorption from bacterial overgrowth and from bypass of the small bowel. Afflicted patients may complain of feculent vomiting or foul-tasting eructation.

Enterovesical fistulas are frequently associated with intra-abdominal abscesses and may present as:

- Dysuria
- Recurrent bladder infections
- Pneumaturia
- Fecaluria.

Vaginal fistulas (rectovaginal or, less often, ileovaginal) may cause dyspareunia or feculent vaginal discharge. A barium enema (after placement of a vaginal tampon) or speculum examination should be diagnostic.

Enterocutaneous fistulas cause intermittent discharge through affected areas of the skin. They most often drain through abdominal surgical scars, following the path of least resistance.

Free perforation, occurring in 1% to 2% of patients, most often occurs in the ileum, while less common sites are the jejunum or a diseased and dilated colon. When perforation occurs, particularly in the case of colonic perforation, the resulting peritonitis may be fatal. Peritonitis may also develop from the rupture of an intra-abdominal abscess.

11

Extraintestinal Manifestations

■ **Skin**

Erythema nodosum is more frequent in Crohn's disease as opposed to pyoderma gangrenosum, which is more common in UC. Aphthous stomatitis is also more common in Crohn's disease and usually shows granulomas when biopsied.

■ **Musculoskeletal**

Clubbing is usually associated with extensive small-bowel disease and correlates with disease activity. Pelvic osteomyelitis can result from fistulization from the small bowel into the pelvic brim and hip joint. Osteomalacia can result from vitamin D and calcium deficiency from either poor oral intake, malabsorption, or corticosteroid use. Steroids, when used chronically, can have deleterious effects on bone, and osteoporosis and aseptic osteonecrosis are well-recognized concerns in steroid-dependent patients.

When Crohn's disease is initially diagnosed or as early as possible into the disease course, bone density should be measured by dual energy x-ray absorptiometry (DEXA) scanning. Management should be based on this initial reading, factoring in the additive risk of osteoporosis from corticosteroid use and any other risk factors that may be present. Surveillance DEXA scans should be checked every year or two, depending on the result of the initial measurement (**Figure 11.3**).

■ **Miscellaneous**

Oxalate kidney stones may result in patients with small-bowel disease who have not had colonic resection. Steatorrhea may promote excessive colonic absorption of oxalate, which is then excreted in the kidneys. Gallstones may be due to changes in the bile-salt pool from either ileal disease or resection and are seen in 15% to 30% of patients with Crohn's disease.

FIGURE 11.3 — MANAGEMENT OF METABOLIC BONE DISEASE IN CROHN'S DISEASE

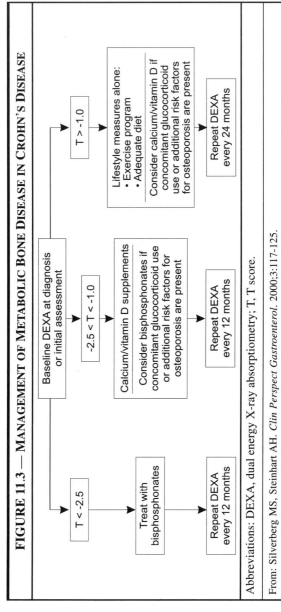

Baseline DEXA at diagnosis or initial assessment

T < -2.5

Treat with bisphosphonates

Repeat DEXA every 12 months

-2.5 < T < -1.0

Calcium/vitamin D supplements

Consider bisphosphonates if concomitant glucocorticoid use or additional risk factors for osteoporosis are present

Repeat DEXA every 12 months

T > -1.0

Lifestyle measures alone:
• Exercise program
• Adequate diet

Consider calcium/vitamin D if concomitant glucocorticoid use or additional risk factors for osteoporosis are present

Repeat DEXA every 24 months

Abbreviations: DEXA, dual energy X-ray absorptiometry; T, T score.

From: Silverberg MS, Steinhart AH. *Clin Perspect Gastroenterol.* 2000;3:117-125.

11

Medication may cause side effects. Sulfasalazine may decrease folate absorption or cause a mild chronic hemolysis, resulting in folate deficiency. Pancreatitis has been reported as a complication of treatment with sulfasalazine, mesalamine, azathioprine, or 6-MP or from hyperlipidemia in patients receiving lipid emulsions as a component of total parenteral nutrition (TPN). Steroid side effects include impaired vitamin D metabolism, effects on bone from impaired calcium transport, and increased delivery of calcium to the urinary tract.

Amyloidosis is rare but can be life threatening, particularly when it involves the kidneys. Presentation usually includes the nephrotic syndrome, but other organs may be affected, including the heart, bowel, liver, spleen, and thyroid. It generally does not respond to treatment of IBD.

Thromboembolic complications include thrombosis of either the lower-extremity or pelvic veins. A stroke may occur in young patients who have no prior evidence of vascular disease. These complications are typically associated with severe disease, particularly colitis.

The most common hepatobiliary manifestations include a fatty liver and primary sclerosing cholangitis (PSC). PSC is more often associated with UC (see Chapter 10, *Ulcerative Colitis*).

Diagnosis

The differential diagnosis of common symptoms and signs of Crohn's disease is shown in **Table 11.2**. An algorithm for the diagnosis of Crohn's disease in adults is shown in **Figure 11.4**.

Stool testing is necessary to:

- Rule out enteric pathogens (eg, *Salmonella*, *Shigella*, *Campylobacter* species, and *Escherichia coli*)

- Check for ova and parasites (using three separate specimens)
- Diagnose *Clostridium difficile* infection.

Radiologic testing that may be helpful in diagnosing Crohn's disease includes several options. Barium studies may show areas of stenosis, fistulas, and inflammatory changes. A small-bowel series or enteroclysis (small-bowel enema) is useful in evaluating symptoms in established disease. Enteroclysis is more detailed in confirming or excluding the diagnosis for the first time, while a small-bowel series is as good or better for detecting complications in established disease. A double-contrast barium enema may demonstrate colitis, terminal ileitis, or fistulas. An ultrasound evaluation (either transabdominal or transrectal), computed tomography (CT) scanning, or magnetic resonance imaging may show abscesses or other masses. Endoscopy is useful in evaluating the extent and location of inflammatory changes. It helps to evaluate and biopsy radiographically abnormal areas, such as filling defects, strictures, and fistulas. Biopsies are needed to firmly establish a primary diagnosis of Crohn's disease. They also help to distinguish Crohn's disease from UC, rule out acute self-limited infectious colitis, and rule out dysplasia or cancer during screening or in evaluation of an abnormal area.

■ Exacerbating Factors

Intercurrent infections may exacerbate Crohn's disease, particularly respiratory tract infections and *C difficile* colitis. Cigarette smoking may cause symptoms to appear, and nonsteroidal anti-inflammatory drugs can aggravate inflammatory bowel disease (IBD) or cause a colitis that mimics it.

TABLE 11.2 — DIFFERENTIAL DIAGNOSIS OF COMMON SYMPTOMS AND SIGNS OF CROHN'S DISEASE

- Acute appendicitis:
  - No chronic bowel symptoms typical of ileitis
  - Progression of pain from epigastrium toward RLQ
  - Constipation is more common than is diarrhea
  - Recurrent subacute appendicitis or an appendiceal abscess may cause symptoms for weeks or months, but patients often will recall a specific time when the original episode of acute appendicitis occurred
  - CT scan or ultrasound may be diagnostic or may require laparoscopy or laparotomy
- Cecal diverticulitis; possibly can be diagnosed non-invasively with CT scan, ultrasound, or barium enema
- Tubo-ovarian abnormalities:
  - Pelvic inflammatory disease or an ectopic pregnancy
  - Ovarian cysts or tumors or endometriosis; should be considered in patients with previously diagnosed Crohn's disease who have new RLQ symptoms
- Neoplastic intestinal disease:
  - Carcinoma of the cecum; may extend into terminal ileum
  - Carcinoid tumor of the ileum or appendix
  - Lymphosarcoma of the jejunum, ileum, or cecum
  - Metastatic carcinoma or melanoma may involve the ileum or cecum
- Ischemic ileitis
- Systemic vasculitis; may cause ulceration, necrosis, hemorrhage, and perforation of the small bowel:
  - Polyarteritis nodosa
  - Systemic lupus erythematosus
  - Rheumatoid arthritis
  - Scleroderma (progressive systemic sclerosis)
  - Necrotizing angiitis
  - Essential mixed cryoglobulinemia
  - Dermatomyositis
  - Behçet's syndrome
- Radiation enteritis
- Intestinal infections/infestations:

- Ileocecal tuberculosis
- Ileocolonic amebiasis (due to *Entamoeba histolytica* infestation)
- Anisakiasis (roundworm found in some raw fish)
- *Yersinia enterocolitica* ileitis
• In patients with AIDS:
  - *Mycobacterium avium-intracellulare* infection
  - Cytomegalovirus infection
• Infiltrative disease of the small bowel or the colon:
  - Eosinophilic gastroenteritis
  - Amyloidosis

Abbreviations: RLQ, right lower quadrant; CT, computed tomography; AIDS, acquired immunodeficiency syndrome.

■ Determining Disease Activity

There are subjective clinical parameters to help determine disease activity, such as the ability to avoid steroids and the avoidance of surgery. Systemic and extraintestinal manifestations also help to determine the activity of the disease. Impact of the disease on the quality of life of the patient should be considered. The Crohn's Disease Activity Index is based on:

• Number of liquid stools per day
• Extent of abdominal pain
• General sense of well-being
• Occurrence of extraintestinal symptoms
• Need for antidiarrheal drugs
• Presence of abdominal masses
• Hematocrit
• Body weight.

■ Working Definitions of Clinical Disease Activity

Mild-to-moderate disease activity is described as:

• Ambulatory patient
• Tolerates an oral diet
• Absence of:
  - Dehydration

183

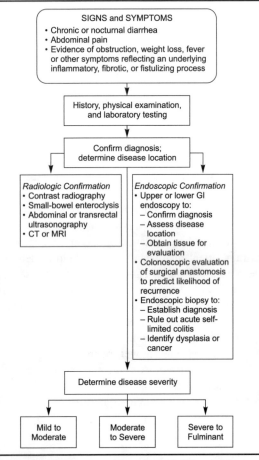

FIGURE 11.4 — DIAGNOSIS OF CROHN'S DISEASE IN ADULTS

SIGNS and SYMPTOMS
- Chronic or nocturnal diarrhea
- Abdominal pain
- Evidence of obstruction, weight loss, fever or other symptoms reflecting an underlying inflammatory, fibrotic, or fistulizing process

↓

History, physical examination, and laboratory testing

↓

Confirm diagnosis; determine disease location

Radiologic Confirmation
- Contrast radiography
- Small-bowel enteroclysis
- Abdominal or transrectal ultrasonography
- CT or MRI

Endoscopic Confirmation
- Upper or lower GI endoscopy to:
  – Confirm diagnosis
  – Assess disease location
  – Obtain tissue for evaluation
- Colonoscopic evaluation of surgical anastomosis to predict likelihood of recurrence
- Endoscopic biopsy to:
  – Establish diagnosis
  – Rule out acute self-limited colitis
  – Identify dysplasia or cancer

↓

Determine disease severity

| Mild to Moderate | Moderate to Severe | Severe to Fulminant |

Abbreviations: CT, computed tomography; MRI, magnetic resonance imaging; GI, gastrointestinal.

Reprinted with permission of the American College of Gastroenterology. *Keys to the Diagnosis and Treatment of Crohn's Disease in Adults*. American College of Gastroenterology: Arlington, Va; 1997 Annual Meeting; and Hanauer SB, Meyers S. *Am J Gastroenterol.* 1997;92:559-566.

- Toxicity (high fevers, rigors)
- Abdominal tenderness
- Painful mass
- Obstruction.

Moderate-to-severe disease activity is described as:
- Patient failed to respond to treatment of mild-to-moderate disease
- More prominent symptoms, such as:
  - Fever
  - Significant weight loss (more than 10% of premorbid body weight)
  - Abdominal pain or tenderness (without rebound)
  - Intermittent nausea or vomiting (without obstruction)
  - Significant anemia.

Severe-to-fulminant disease activity is described as:
- Persistent symptoms despite outpatient use of corticosteroids
- More significant symptoms such as:
  - High fever
  - Persistent vomiting
  - Evidence of intestinal obstruction
  - Rebound tenderness
  - Cachexia
  - Evidence of an abscess.

Remission is described as:
- Asymptomatic or without inflammatory sequelae such as fistulae or abscesses
- Responded to medical intervention
- Completion of surgical resection without gross residual disease
- Not requiring ongoing use of corticosteroids.

11

Management

Goals of treatment in Crohn's disease are to:
- Maintain symptomatic control
- Optimize quality of life
- Minimize short- and long-term toxicity of therapy
- Delay or reduce likelihood of recurrence after surgery.

A management algorithm for Crohn's disease in adults is shown in **Figure 11.5**. Many of the medications used in the management of Crohn's disease are the same as those used in UC and are described in detail in Chapter 10, *Ulcerative Colitis*. Aminosalicylates or antibiotics are the first-line agents used in milder disease, while corticosteroids are reserved for unresponsive disease, more severe flares, or inflammatory complications. Immunomodulators, including azathioprine and 6-mercaptopurine (6-MP) play a role in managing yet more severe flares. These medications should be considered when corticosteroid side effects are intolerable or when a reduction in steroid dosage cannot be accomplished otherwise. In some instances, immunomodulators may be the only medications successful in achieving or maintaining a clinical remission. Methotrexate may be useful as a steroid-sparing drug and appears to be more effective in achieving an early remission in Crohn's disease than in UC. Cyclosporine A is ineffective in managing acute flares or maintaining remission, but it may be useful in fistulous disease. Omega-3 fatty acids have an as yet undefined role in treating active Crohn's colitis.

As is the case with UC, the need for treatment of Crohn's disease is primarily based on symptoms and documented complications, rather than on the endoscopic appearance of the bowel. Practice guidelines are classified according to severity of the disease and subdivided into acute and maintenance phases (Hanauer and Meyers, 1997).

■ **Acute Flare**
Mild-to-Moderate Disease

Treatment for mild-to-moderate ileal, ileocolonic, or colonic disease includes:

- Oral aminosalicylates: Sulfasalazine 3 to 6 g/day divided bid, tid or qid, or mesalamine 2000 to 4800 mg/day po divided tid or qid; effective in achieving remission in 50% of cases and can be continued at the same or smaller dose for maintenance of remission. These agents are more effective in colonic than in small-bowel disease, although mesalamine (Pentasa) is active in the small intestine. Sulfasalazine is far less expensive than newer aminosalicylates, but the likelihood of intolerance due to side effects is much greater with sulfasalazine.

- Oral budesonide (Entocort EC): Budesonide is an oral corticosteroid with negligible systemic absorption that is effective in ileal and ascending colonic Crohn's disease. The active agent is protected from gastric acid in granules that dissolve at pH >5.5 (in the duodenum). Thereafter, breakdown of the matrix of ethylcellulose and budesonide releases the active drug by a time-release mechanism. After absorption, first-pass metabolism of 80% to 90% of the drug by the liver results in two inactive metabolites. The usual dose is 9 mg (three 3-mg capsules) once each morning for up to 8 weeks. Recurrent Crohn's flares can also be treated with a similar 8-week course.

- Antibiotics: Metronidazole 10 to 20 mg/kg/day or 1 to 2 g/day for 3 to 6 months; may help a subset of patients who have not responded to or cannot tolerate oral aminosalicylate therapy.

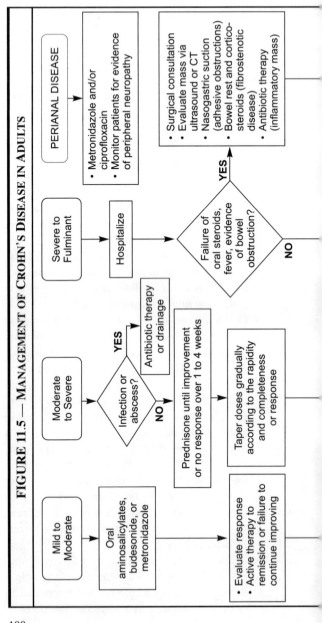

FIGURE 11.5 — MANAGEMENT OF CROHN'S DISEASE IN ADULTS

PERIANAL DISEASE
- Metronidazole and/or ciprofloxacin
- Monitor patients for evidence of peripheral neuropathy

Severe to Fulminant → Hospitalize

Failure of oral steroids, fever, evidence of bowel obstruction?

YES:
- Surgical consultation
- Evaluate mass via ultrasound or CT
- Nasogastric suction (adhesive obstructions)
- Bowel rest and corticosteroids (fibrostenotic disease)
- Antibiotic therapy (inflammatory mass)

NO

Moderate to Severe

Infection or abscess?

YES → Antibiotic therapy or drainage

NO → Prednisone until improvement or no response over 1 to 4 weeks

Taper doses gradually according to the rapidity and completeness or response

Mild to Moderate → Oral aminosalicylates, budesonide, or metronidazole

- Evaluate response
- Active therapy to remission or failure to continue improving

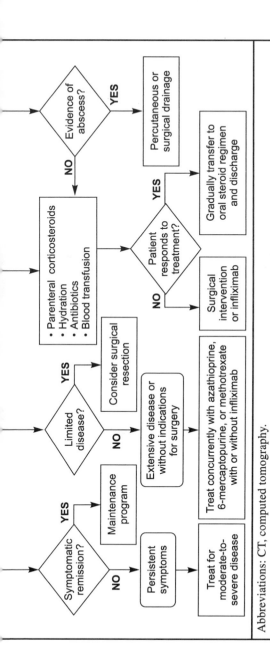

Abbreviations: CT, computed tomography.

Adapted from : American College of Gastroenterology. *Keys to the Diagnosis and Treatment of Crohn's Disease in Adults*. American College of Gastroenterology: Arlington, Va; 1997 Annual Meeting; and Hanauer SB, Meyers S. *Am J Gastroenterol*. 1997;92:559-566.

Long-term use (more than 3 to 4 months) is often required but may be complicated by a debilitating peripheral neuropathy. In addition to its antibacterial properties, metronidazole interferes directly with the inflammatory process. It is equal in efficacy to aminosalicylates in the management of acute Crohn's colitis and is especially useful in perianal and perineal complications such as perianal fistulae. It is also effective in treatment of *C difficile* infection, which may occasionally be responsible for a flare of IBD. Ciprofloxacin or clarithromycin may be a better-tolerated substitute for metronidazole, or they can be used in combination with it for perianal disease.

Mild-to-moderate gastroduodenal Crohn's disease may respond to acid suppression, by H_2-receptor antagonists (cimetidine, ranitidine, famotidine, or nizatidine) or by proton pump inhibitors (omeprazole or lansoprazole). 6-MP has been used in refractory cases.

Jejunoileitis is often complicated by small-bowel bacterial overgrowth and may respond best to antibiotic agents such as tetracycline or ciprofloxacin.

Moderate-to-Severe Disease
Once infection and abscess (which require drainage with or without surgery) are excluded, several treatment steps may be taken. Elemental diets may be effective in some patients. Pharmacologic therapy includes:
- Corticosteroids: prednisone 40 to 60 mg/day or methylprednisolone 0.5 to 0.75 mg/kg/day. This regimen is used until symptoms resolve and weight gain resumes. The full dose should be used until symptoms respond well, often taking

7 to 28 days; then the dose should be tapered as follows:
– Decrease by 5 to 10 mg/day until dose is 20 mg/day;
– Then decrease by 2.5 to 5 mg/day until discontinuation is possible.

There is no benefit to adding an oral aminosalicylate to the steroid acutely. Because nearly half of these patients will become steroid dependent or resistant, surgical resection should be considered in limited disease. In extensive disease or if there is no indication for surgery, 6-MP (Purinethol) or azathioprine (Imuran) can be added in refractory disease. Elemental diets by mouth, via feeding tubes into the stomach or jejunum, or regular full liquid diets may be equivalent and of value.

Infliximab (Remicade) is a monoclonal antibody that binds to and inhibits the functional activity of tumor necrosis factor-alpha (TNF-α). It is useful in moderate-to-severe Crohn's disease for which conventional therapy has failed or at times as a bridge for more rapid control of disease until 6-MP, azathioprine, or methotrexate becomes effective. Fistulizing disease is particularly responsive to infliximab. Other potential indications are shown in **Table 11.3**. Patients with congestive heart failure or active infection should not be treated with this medication, and caution should be used in individuals with latent tuberculosis, other chronic or recurrent infections, and some neurologic diseases.

A single induction dose of 5 mg/kg body weight has shown efficacy in active Crohn's disease or when fistulae are present. However, because of the relapsing nature of Crohn's disease, patients will generally require both induction and maintenance therapy. This is indicated to maintain improvement or remission in

TABLE 11.3 — DEFINITE AND POTENTIAL TREATMENT INDICATIONS FOR USE OF INFLIXIMAB IN PATIENTS WITH INFLAMMATORY BOWEL DISEASE

Definite Indications for Induction Therapy
- Moderate-to-severe inflammatory Crohn's disease with an inadequate response to conventional therapy (defined by severity of symptoms and/or lack of response to standard therapy such as corticosteroids, azathioprine, 6-mercaptopurine, and methotrexate)
- Fistulizing Crohn's disease with draining enterocutaneous or perianal fistulas

Potential Indications for Induction Therapy
- Hospitalized patients with inflammatory or fistulizing Crohn's disease who have not failed all conventional therapies where there is either a severe clinical presentation or a rapid onset of action is desired
- Pediatric Crohn's disease
- Steroid-treated Crohn's disease (a form of maintenance therapy)
- Other manifestations of Crohn's disease (Crohn's disease of the ileoanal pouch, ankylosing spondylitis and sacroiliitis, pyoderma gangrenosum, Crohn's disease–associated arthritis, metastatic and perineal-wound Crohn's disease, orofacial Crohn's disease, esophageal Crohn's disease)
- Moderate-to-severe ulcerative colitis unresponsive to conventional therapy
- Severe, steroid-refractory ulcerative colitis

Definite Indications for Maintenance Therapy
- Inflammatory or fistulizing Crohn's disease that responds to initial induction therapy with infliximab and failed maintenance therapy with one or more immunosuppressive agents
- Steroid-treated Crohn's disease that failed an attempt at steroid sparing with one or more immunosuppressive agents

Sandborn WJ, et al. *Am J Gastroenterol.* 2002;97:2962-2972.

patients who previously had moderate-to-severe inflammatory or fistulous disease and in whom other therapy failed. This is an effective means of avoiding steroids (either prednisone or budesonide), which should be discontinued once infliximab, 6-MP, azathioprine, or methotrexate is therapeutic. A maintenance dose of 5 to 10 mg/kg should be used, with the exact dose being based on the duration of benefit of the first maintenance dose, and at least three doses are generally administered. Single-dose therapy or too long an interval between doses of infliximab seems to increase the likelihood of hypersensitivity reactions or to promote the development of human antichimeric antibodies (HACA), thus the FDA has approved a dosing schedule of 5 mg/kg given at 0, 2, and 6 weeks. A single infusion tends to provide benefit for 8 to 12 weeks in many patients, thus a maintenance dose is typically given every 8 weeks.

Azathioprine, 6-MP, or methotrexate is typically prescribed in combination with infliximab, unless a patient has demonstrated intolerance to these immunosuppressant drugs. This combination decreases the immunogenecity of infliximab and reduces formation of antinuclear and anti–double-stranded antibodies that may result in a drug-induced lupuslike syndrome.

Reactivation of latent tuberculosis has been reported in a number of individuals, leading to the recommendation that all patients who are to receive infliximab should first have purified protein derivative (PPD) skin testing. If there is evidence of tuberculosis, this must be treated before initiating infliximab therapy.

Severe-to-Fulminant Disease

Hospitalization is typically required for severe-to-fulminant disease. Surgical evaluation is needed if an obstruction is found or if the patient has a tender abdominal mass, although obstruction due to inflammation may respond to medical therapy alone. Abdominal masses should be evaluated by ultrasound or CT scan to rule out an abscess and, if found, should be treated with percutaneous or open surgical drainage, along with antibiotics.

If the patient has been taking prednisone 40 to 60 mg/day po and an abscess has been excluded, yet symptoms have persisted or worsened, parenteral corticosteroids should be instituted. Doses equivalent to prednisone 40 to 60 mg/day, either continuously or in divided doses (eg, methylprednisolone, 32 to 48 mg/day) are appropriate.

Enteral nutritional support, orally or by tube, may be useful. Parenteral nutrition or an elemental diet is only indicated if an oral diet is intolerable and if nutritional support would be required for more than 5 to 7 days. Supplemental fluids and electrolytes are used as needed in dehydrated patients.

Oral feedings are acceptable if tolerated and the patient has neither severe abdominal pain nor an obstruction. Bowel rest and IV nutrition are needed if an obstruction from inflammation, fibrotic stricturing, or adhesion, or severe clinical toxicity is present. Broad-spectrum antibiotic therapy is warranted in the event of inflammatory strictures. Oral steroids can be resumed if the patient responds well.

Perianal disease usually responds to metronidazole or, if necessary, another antibiotic such as ciprofloxacin. Metronidazole is prescribed at a dose of 10 to 20 mg/kg/day in divided doses. Long-term use (more than 3 to 4 months) is often required but may be complicated by peripheral neuropathy that can be quite debilitating. For this reason, other agents such as immunosuppressives or infliximab may need to be utilized if a protracted course of metronidazole would otherwise be necessary..

Maintenance Therapy

Most patients should remain on medication continuously and indefinitely as relapses may thus be prevented or delayed. Withdrawal of azathioprine or 6-MP may be safe after 4 years of steady remission; however, this is still under study. Corticosteroids are not effective in this setting and should not be used to maintain patients in clinical remission, although patients who are steroid-dependent (ie, who become symptomatic below a certain dose) appear to benefit from continuation.

Azathioprine 2.5 mg/kg/day or 6-MP 1.5 mg/kg/day (or until mild leukopenia is observed) may help to reduce necessary steroid doses. Therapy for 3 to 6 months is often required before effectiveness may be recognized. The blood count should be periodically monitored since leukopenia may be delayed and severe. Pancreatitis may occur in up to 15% of patients taking azathioprine or 6-MP.

Methotrexate, 25 mg intramuscularly or subcutaneously weekly, is also effective in reducing steroid requirements. It has not been studied in comparison with 6-MP or azathioprine, however.

Mesalamine at doses >3 g/day may be useful in maintenance of remission and in preventing recurrence after resection for Crohn's disease.

Indications for Surgery

Surgery is eventually required in up to 66% of patients because of:
- Massive hemorrhage
- Perforation
- Persistent or recurrent obstruction
- Suppurative complications, including intra-abdominal or pelvic abscesses
- Medically intractable disease (unresponsive fulminant disease) or toxic megacolon

195

- Intolerable side effects from medication (eg, steroid dependence or peripheral neuropathy from metronidazole)
- Failure to respond to 7 to 10 days of intensive inpatient management
- Malignancy (when resectable).

"Neither patients nor physicians should view surgery as a sign of failure. It is an effective therapy that often proves to be the swiftest, safest and most effective route to physical and psychosocial rehabilitation." (Hanauer and Meyers, 1997.)

Surgical Procedures

■ Colorectal or Ileal Crohn's Disease

Surgical options for colorectal or ileal Crohn's disease include:

- Subtotal colectomy (leaving the rectum *in situ*) and ileostomy:
  - Most often used in toxic colitis, toxic megacolon, and high-risk surgical patients who require colectomy but may not tolerate proctectomy
  - Completion proctectomy is often required after the patient's condition is stabilized
- End ileostomy without colonic resection:
  - Usually done as a temporary measure in patients with perianal sepsis or a rectovaginal or other pelvic fistula who require fecal diversion
  - Can be used in the management of toxic megacolon in high-risk patients, such as pregnant or elderly persons
  - Can serve as a preliminary procedure in patients who will require proctocolectomy but who are too ill to tolerate that operation in one step

- Can be performed laparoscopically in some patients
- Total proctocolectomy and ileostomy:
  - Surgical procedure of choice in extensive Crohn's colitis associated with significant anorectal inflammation
  - Indicated when colectomy is required and anal sphincter function is poor
  - Proctectomy is done as part of a single procedure or may need to be delayed if there is serious perianal disease
- Abdominal colectomy and ileorectal anastomosis:
  - Utilized when there is extensive colitis but the rectum is unaffected and there is good anal sphincter function
  - Can be done as a two-step procedure in which colectomy and end ileostomy are followed by ileorectal anastomosis when the comorbid condition or conditions that delayed this step have resolved or in a single combined operation
  - Fecal incontinence may be a problem if ileitis or proctitis ensue subsequent to surgery
  - Contraindications: active perianal disease, rectal cancer or dysplasia, or a poorly compliant rectum
- Ileocolonic disease can be excised with an ileocolonic anastomosis, ideally with 5-cm disease-free margins at each end of the resected specimen
- Multiple ileal strictures:
  - If closely spaced, can be resected *en bloc*
  - If widely separated, options are to do separate stricturoplasties (**Figure 11.6**) or to bypass affected segments of diseased ileum with side-to-side anastomoses between healthy segments of ileum and adjacent colon
  - Stricturoplasty is most effective if short strictures encompass a long segment of ileum in

11

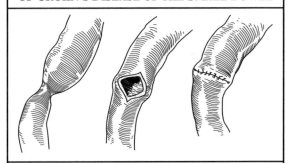
patients who have had prior small-bowel re-
sections and for fibrotic rather than acute inflammatory strictures.

An ileoanal anastomosis is highly problematic in
Crohn's disease because of the frequency of anal and
perianal manifestations of the disease, but a number of
patients thought preoperatively to have UC (until their
colectomy specifically showed Crohn's disease) have
tolerated it well in some series. Continent ileostomies
are rarely performed; however, patients who have been
free of symptoms and have not required steroids for at
least 5 years may do well with this procedure.

■ Colonic Fistulas

Ileosigmoid fistulas can be managed with an ileocecal resection and ileocolonic anastomosis, combined

with a segmental sigmoid resection and colocolic anastomosis. Fistulas to the urinary bladder from the ileum, sigmoid, or rectum usually require an ileal or colonic resection but typically do not require formal bladder excision. The defect in the bladder can either be left open, excised locally then closed, or closed primarily.

■ Enteroenteric Fistulas

These fistulas are often treated with medication and possibly with enteral or parenteral nutritional support; however, if conservative therapy proves ineffective, segmental resections at each point of the fistula with primary enteroenterostomies can be performed.

SUGGESTED READING

Bickston SJ, Cominelli F. Treatment of Crohn's disease at the turn of the century. *N Engl J Med*. 1998;339:401-402. Editorial.

Fazio VW, Wu JS. Surgical therapy for Crohn's disease of the colon and rectum. *Surg Clin North Am*. 1997;77:197-210.

Hanauer SB, Meyers S. Management of Crohn's disease in adults. *Am J Gastroenterol*. 1997;92:559-566.

Sands BE. Crohn's disease. In: Feldman M, Friedman LS, Sleisenger MH, eds. *Sleisenger and Fordtran's Gastrointestinal and Liver Disease*: *Pathophysiology/Diagnosis/Management*. 7th ed. Philadelphia, Pa: WB Saunders Co; 2002:2005-2038.

Sandborn WJ, Hanauer SB. Infliximab in the treatment of Crohn's disease: a user's guide for clinicians. *Am J Gastroenterol*. 2002;97:2962-2972.

12 Epidemiology and Biology of Colorectal Cancer

Incidence and Prevalence

Colorectal cancer (CRC) accounts for 10% of cancer deaths, second only to lung cancer in the United States. In 2003, there were an estimated 147,000 new cases and 51,000 deaths from CRC. The cumulative lifetime risk is approximately 6%.

In the United States, geographic distribution favors the mid-Atlantic states, New England, and population centers in the Midwest. The age-adjusted incidence and mortality rates for CRC have decreased over the past 50 years, possibly due to (**Figure 12.1**):

- Earlier detection
- More accurate diagnosis
- More effective treatment.

Clinical Features

Colorectal cancer is predominately a disease of people 50 years of age and older (**Figure 12.2**). The overall 5-year survival rate is:

- White males — 61%
- White females — 59%
- Black males — 48%
- Black females — 49%.

Adenomatous polyps and CRC can occur throughout the colon and rectum, with 50% occurring proximal to the splenic flexure (**Figure 12.3**).

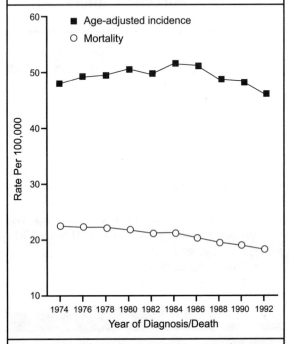

FIGURE 12.1 — AGE-ADJUSTED INCIDENCE AND MORTALITY OF COLORECTAL CANCER IN THE GENERAL POPULATION OVER TIME

- ■ Age-adjusted incidence
- ○ Mortality

Rate Per 100,000

Year of Diagnosis/Death

Adapted from: Ries LA, et al. *SEER Cancer Statistic Review, 1973-1991*. Bethesda, Md: 1994.

Polyps

Polyps are mucosal masses that occur in the colon and rectum (**Figure 12.4**). Adenomatous polyps (adenomas) are premalignant and account for about two thirds of polyps. Hyperplastic polyps, mucosal tags, lipomas, and hamartomas probably have no clinical importance.

By age 50 years, 25% of people have adenomas (**Figure 12.5**). This increases to over 50% of people

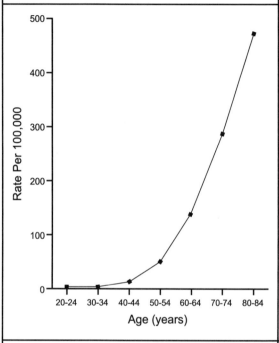

FIGURE 12.2 — AGE-SPECIFIC INCIDENCE OF COLORECTAL CANCER IN THE GENERAL POPULATION

Adapted from: Ries LA, et al. *SEER Cancer Statistic Review, 1973-1991*. Bethesda, Md: 1994.

12

at age 80. Adenomas are distributed in the bowel in the following approximate percentages:

- Rectosigmoid — 50%
- Ascending colon and cecum — 20%
- Descending colon — 18%
- Transverse colon — 11%.

High-grade dysplasia is likely to occur in 1% of adenomas <5 mm, 5% of 5-mm to 9-mm adenomas and 20% of adenomas >1 cm. Patients with adenomas

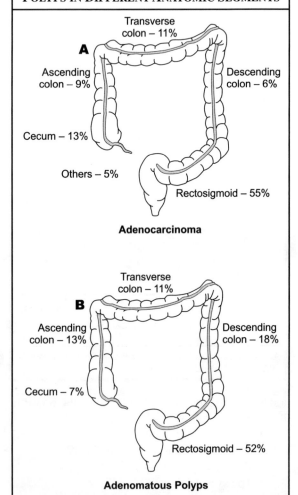

FIGURE 12.3 — FREQUENCY OF ADENOCARCINOMA AND ADENOMATOUS POLYPS IN DIFFERENT ANATOMIC SEGMENTS

A

Transverse colon – 11%

Ascending colon – 9%

Descending colon – 6%

Cecum – 13%

Others – 5%

Rectosigmoid – 55%

Adenocarcinoma

B

Transverse colon – 11%

Ascending colon – 13%

Descending colon – 18%

Cecum – 7%

Rectosigmoid – 52%

Adenomatous Polyps

Adapted from: Winawer SJ, Enker WE, Levin B. Colorectal cancer. In: Winawaer SJ, ed. *Management of Gastrointestinal Diseases*. New York, NY: Gower Medical; 1992.

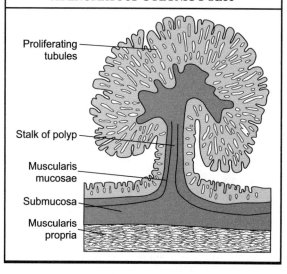

FIGURE 12.4 — CROSS-SECTIONAL REPRESENTATION OF ADENOMATOUS COLONIC POLYP

Proliferating tubules

Stalk of polyp

Muscularis mucosae

Submucosa

Muscularis propria

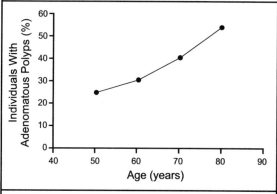

FIGURE 12.5 — PREVALENCE OF ADENOMATOUS POLYPS BY AGE IN THE GENERAL POPULATION

Individuals With Adenomatous Polyps (%)

Age (years)

Adapted from: Winawer SJ, et al. *Gastroenterology*. 1997;112: 594-642.

12

larger than 1 cm are three times more likely to develop CRC than the general population, and patients with multiple adenomas are six times more likely to develop CRC (**Figures 12.6 and 12.7**).

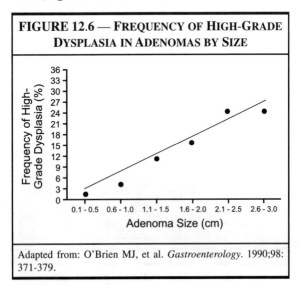

FIGURE 12.6 — FREQUENCY OF HIGH-GRADE DYSPLASIA IN ADENOMAS BY SIZE

Adapted from: O'Brien MJ, et al. *Gastroenterology*. 1990;98: 371-379.

Few adenomas develop into cancer; the rate of transformation is estimated to be 2.5 polyps/1000/y. It is estimated, based on observational studies and case control studies, that it takes an average of 10 years for an adenoma <1 cm to transform into an invasive cancer.

There is a relationship between adenomatous polyps in siblings and the risk for a patient to develop colon cancer in his/her lifetime. **Figure 12.7** shows that an individual with a family history of polyps in siblings before age 50 greatly increases the risk of developing CRC by age 55. If the individual has a sibling with polyps diagnosed between ages 50 and 59 years, the risk is intermediate and the shift in time of occurrence of the colon cancer is more toward age 60

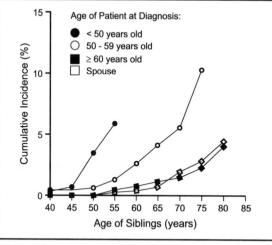

FIGURE 12.7 — CUMULATIVE INCIDENCE OF COLORECTAL CANCER IN SIBLINGS OF PATIENTS WITH ADENOMAS

Age of Patient at Diagnosis:
● < 50 years old
○ 50 - 59 years old
■ ≥ 60 years old
□ Spouse

Adapted from: Winawer SJ, et al. *Gastroenterology*. 1997;112: 594-642.

to 65. The figure also shows that the individual has a normal risk for developing cancer if the polyps are identified in the sibling after 60 years of age. These data from the National Polyp Study, therefore, show that both adenomatous polyps and cancer are inherited and must be considered as a single disease entity.

As shown in **Figure 12.8**, there is an orderly progression from the normal colon mucosa to the small adenoma to a larger adenoma and finally an adenoma with high-grade dysplasia leading to invasive adenocarcinoma. Because the high-grade dysplasia and early adenocarcinoma may ulcerate, the tumor at the time of diagnosis no longer resembles a polypoid growth but rather may be flat, ulcerated, and invasive, with constriction of the surrounding bowel.

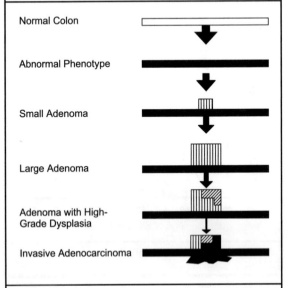

FIGURE 12.8 — SCHEMATIC OUTLINE OF THE EVOLUTION OF COLORECTAL CARCINOMA FROM THE NORMAL MUCOSA

Normal Colon

Abnormal Phenotype

Small Adenoma

Large Adenoma

Adenoma with High-Grade Dysplasia

Invasive Adenocarcinoma

Adapted from: O'Brien MJ, et al. *Cancer*. 1992;70(suppl 5): 1317-1327.

Pathogenesis of Colorectal Cancer

The human diet has been linked to bowel cancer etiology since Dennis Burkett made his seminal observation that CRC, diverticular disease, and constipation are rare among native Africans who eat a diet high in vegetable fiber and low in animal fat. More recently, meta-analysis of 13 case-controlled studies shows an inverse relationship of CRC mortality with high consumption of vegetable and/or cereal fiber. Diets high in animal meat/fat are associated with increased CRC rates.

The illustration in **Figure 12.9** compares and contrasts the effect of fat and fiber on the metabolic activity of the large bowel and suggests ways in which bowel cancer might be enhanced or inhibited. Dietary fat leads to bile acids and liposoluble toxic chemicals, which produce an alkaline pH, an overgrowth of anaerobic bacteria and bile-acid degradation, to cause nitrosamine formation. Fat in the diet is a source of diacylglycerol (DAG), which promotes activation of K-*ras* oncogene and cell turnover. Furthermore, charcooking fatty meat at high temperature produces high levels of intraluminal heterocyclic amines, which are also carcinogenic.

On the other hand, dietary fiber reaches the large bowel essentially undigested where it binds to bile ac-

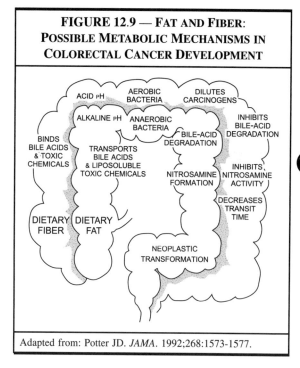

FIGURE 12.9 — FAT AND FIBER: POSSIBLE METABOLIC MECHANISMS IN COLORECTAL CANCER DEVELOPMENT

Adapted from: Potter JD. *JAMA.* 1992;268:1573-1577.

ids and other toxic chemicals, and produces an acid pH and aerobic bacteria growth, which inhibits bile acid degradation. The undigested dietary fiber dilutes carcinogens, inhibits nitrosamine activity, and speeds up the transit time in the bowel. In addition, diets high in calcium also bind bile acids and fatty acids in the large bowel, thereby reducing exposure to potential carcinogenic compounds.

At the cellular level, scientists have shown that the basal cells of the bowel crypts are epithelial stem cells, which when stimulated overgrow the crypt to give rise to aberrant crypts and ultimately adenomatous polyps (**Figure 12.10**). Biopsies of the large bowel can be used to demonstrate aberrant crypts and abnormal proliferation as a cellular marker in individuals who are at increased risk for large-bowel cancer.

At the molecular level, Vogelstein and colleagues postulated that a series of genetic mutations are associated with progression of the dysplastic polyp to invasive colorectal carcinoma (**Figure 12.11**):

- Hypomethylated DNA
- K-*ras* mutation on chromosome 12p
- DCC loss on chromosome 18q
- p53 loss on chromosome 17p.

In addition to the mutations that are associated with progression of invasive CRC, several mutations are inherited which are permissive or increase the likelihood of CRC developing in family members:

- APC gene mutations result in hundreds of adenomatous polyps in the familial adenomatous polyp syndrome.
- Mismatch repair gene mutations (h-MLH-1, h-MSH-2) facilitate mutation rate in hereditary nonpolyposis colon cancer (HNPCC) patients.
- In juvenile polyposis syndrome and ulcerative colitis, stromal proliferation stimulates carcinoma formation.

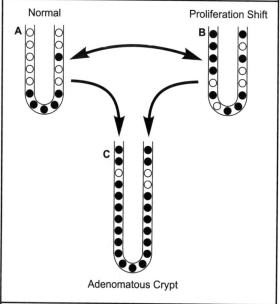

FIGURE 12.10 — SCHEMATIC DEMONSTRATION OF CHANGES IN EPITHELIAL CELL PROLIFERATION OF ADENOMATOUS TRANSFORMATION OF THE MUCOSAL CRYPT

Normal

Proliferation Shift

A

B

C

Adenomatous Crypt

(A) In the normal crypt, proliferating cells (dark circles) are confined largely to the lower 33% of the crypt. (B) Abnormal proliferation is seen where more than 50% of the proliferating cells of the crypt are located in the mid and upper 33%. (C) In an adenomatous crypt, there is morphologic change, dysplastic nuclei, and elongation, with or without branching, in addition to abnormal proliferation.

Adapted from: O'Brien MJ, et al. *Cancer.* 1992;70(suppl 5): 1317-1327.

12

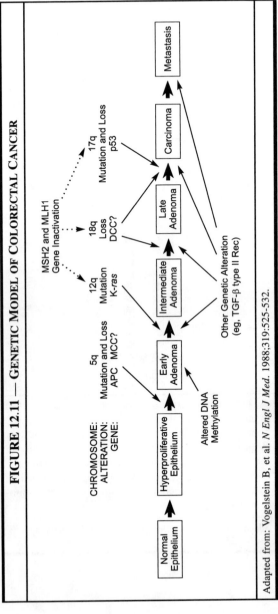

FIGURE 12.11 — GENETIC MODEL OF COLORECTAL CANCER

Adapted from: Vogelstein B, et al. *N Engl J Med.* 1988;319:525-532.

Risk of Colorectal Cancer

About 75% of all new cases of CRC occur in people with no known predisposing factors. People with a family history of CRC but no apparent genetic syndrome make up 15% to 20% of the new cases of CRC. When the individual is a member of a family with a genetic syndrome predisposing to colon cancer, the risk of colon cancer as shown in **Figure 12.12** approaches 100% by age 60 for familial adenomatous polyposis (FAP) subjects and nearly 50% by age 65 for HNPCC subjects. In contrast, the risk of colon cancer in the general population is about 4% to 6% by age 65.

Familial adenomatous polyposis accounts for about 1% of annual new cases of CRC. FAP is associated with the mutation of the APC gene located on the long arm of chromosome 5, which is inherited as an

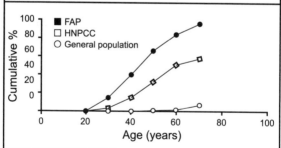

FIGURE 12.12 — CUMULATIVE INCIDENCE OF COLORECTAL CANCER BY AGE IN SUBJECTS WITH GENETIC SYNDROMES COMPARED WITH GENERAL POPULATION

Abbreviations: FAP, familial adenomatous polyposis; HNPCC, hereditary nonpolyposis colon cancer.

Adapted from: Winawer SJ, et al. *Gastroenterology.* 1997;112: 594-642.

autosomal-dominant syndrome. Affected individuals characteristically develop hundreds or thousands of adenomatous polyps in the colon by age 30 and have an almost 100% chance of developing CRC by age 40. Variations of FAP include Turcot's syndrome (familial CRC and brain cancer) and Gardner's syndrome (familial CRC, osteomas, and benign soft tissue tumors). Affected individuals should have a total colectomy by age 30 years to reduce the risk of CRC.

Hereditary nonpolyposis colon cancer, or Lynch Syndrome Type I, accounts for about 5% of new CRC cases in the United States. As shown in **Figure 12.13**, the hereditary nature of this syndrome may be difficult to diagnose. The kindred shown also emphasize that penetration of the gene from one generation to the next may be incomplete. CRC occurs in the fourth and fifth decades, predominantly in the right or proximal colon (**Table 12.1**). Adenomatous polyps precede the development of cancer but do not occur in large numbers. HNPCC is associated with other familial cancers, including those of the endometrium, ureter, small bowel, and stomach. Classically, HNPCC is characterized (Amsterdam criteria) by three or more relatives with CRC, one of whom is a first-degree relative; one or more with CRC diagnosed before age 50 years; and CRC cancer in two generations (**Table 12.2**). Cancers from HNPCC carriers show a mutation in mismatch-repair enzymes that produce microsatellite instability or replication-error phenotype. The genetic mutations occur in hMLH-1, hMSH-2, hPMS-1, hPMS-2, which are found on chromosomes 2, 3, and 7. Patients with HNPCC should undergo subtotal colectomy for treatment of adenomas or CRC. Women should be considered for elective bilateral salpingo-oophorectomy and total abdominal hysterectomy.

Inflammatory bowel disease (IBD) is found in patients with long-standing active ulcerative colitis or Crohn's disease; such patients have a 30% cumulative incidence

FIGURE 12.13 — TYPICAL HEREDITARY NONPOLYPOSIS COLON CANCER KINDRED

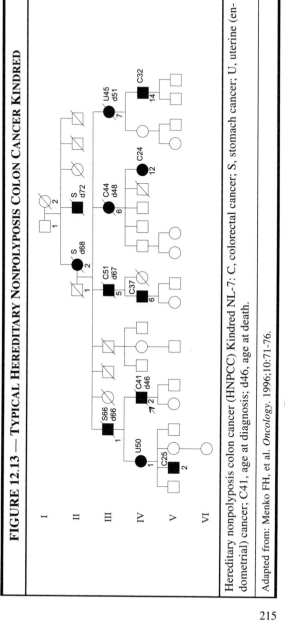

Hereditary nonpolyposis colon cancer (HNPCC) Kindred NL-7: C, colorectal cancer; S, stomach cancer; U, uterine (endometrial) cancer; C41, age at diagnosis; d46, age at death.

Adapted from: Menko FH, et al. *Oncology.* 1996;10:71-76.

TABLE 12.1 — CLINICAL CHARACTERISTICS OF HEREDITARY NONPOLYPOSIS COLON CANCER

Patient Characteristics
- Early onset of colorectal cancer (mean age, 40 to 45 years)
- Proximal tumor localization (60% of tumors)
- Multiple primary colorectal cancers
- Extracolonic tumors:
  - Cancer of the endometrium (most frequent)
  - Stomach
  - Small intestine
  - Upper urologic tract (renal pelvis and ureter)
  - Ovary
  - Skin (Muir-Torre syndrome)

Family Characteristics
- Multiple affected family members
- Pattern of autosomal dominant inheritance with a high rate of penetrance (-90%)

Adapted from: Menko FH, et al. *Oncology*. 1996;10:71-76.

TABLE 12.2 — AMSTERDAM CRITERIA FOR IDENTIFICATION OF HEREDITARY NONPOLYPOSIS COLON CANCER

- Histologically confirmed colorectal cancer in at least three relatives, two of whom are a first-degree relative of the other two
- Occurrence of the disease in at least two successive generations
- Age at diagnosis below 50 years in at least one patient
- Exclusion of familial adenomatous polyposis

Adapted from: Menko FH, et al. *Oncology*. 1996;10:71-76.

of CRC in 35 years. IBD accounts for about 1% of new cases of CRC. The pathogenesis of CRC and IBD is not known. Patients with long-standing active IBD should be considered for colectomy.

Patients with a history of CRC are at increased risk to develop another metachronous CRC at about 0.35%/year reaching 6.3% at 18 years. They should have a lifetime surveillance of the large bowel with annual fecal occult blood test (FOBT) and every 3- to 5-year colonoscopy.

Primary Prevention of Colorectal Cancer

As shown in **Table 12.3**, several large randomized trials of colon cancer prevention have been initiated in the United States. All of them utilize patients who have sporadic polyps for entry on study, most using diet or micronutrients as the randomized intervention. The completed trials showed no survival benefit or decrease in polyp formation in the treated compared with the placebo-treated patients.

Dietary factors are considered to be responsible for 85% to 90% of all cases of CRC. Epidemiologic, animal, and biochemical studies suggest that diets high in total calories and fat, as well as low in dietary fiber, vegetables, and micronutrients, are associated with increased CRC incidence (**Table 12.4**). Americans typically receive 35% to 40% of calories from fat; reduction in fat consumption to <25% calories from fat is advocated by the USDA/DHHS. Short-term intervention studies indicate that wheat bran supplementation >10 g/day will decrease the labeling index in bowel crypt cells. Calcium supplements in excess of 1250 mg/day will lower the labeling index in bowel mucosal cells. Folic acid supplements of 400 mg/day are associated in case-control studies with a 50% reduction in CRC incidence.

Investigator/Institution	Patient Population	Randomzied Agent	Outcome
D. Alberts University of Arizona	Sporadic polyps	High vs low wheat bran fiber	No effect
J. Baron (Multicenter) Dartmouth University	Sporadic polyps	Calcium vs placebo	Small reduction in small polyps
J. Baron (Multicenter) Dartmouth University	Sporadic polyps	Aspirin vs placebo	Small reduction in small polyps
R. Greenberg (Multicenter) Dartmouth University	Sporadic polyps	Factorial: Vitamin A, betacarotene, vitamin E	No effect
I. Macrae Melbourne	Sporadic polyps	Factorial: low fat/high fiber/ betacarotene	No effect
A. Schatzkin (Multicenter) National Cancer Institute	Sporadic polyps	Low fat/5.8 servings of fruits and vegetables vs standard diet	No effect

TABLE 12.3 — ONGOING PHASE III TRIAL OF NEW STRATEGIES TO PREVENT THE RECURRENCE OF SPORADIC COLORECTAL ADENOMAS

Adapted from: Vargas PA, Alberts DS. *Cancer.* 1992;70(suppl 5):1229-1235.

TABLE 12.4 — SUMMARY OF EPIDEMIOLOGIC STUDIES: ASSOCIATIONS BETWEEN FIBER-RICH DIETS AND COLON CANCER

Study Type	Number of Studies	Associations*		
		Inverse	None	Direct
International correlation	7	6	1	0
Within country correlation	6	6	0	0
Case control	16	10	4	2
Metabolic	7	6	1	0
Cohort	1	1	0	0
Time trend	3	3	0	0
Total	40	32	6	2

*Associations between fiber intake or fiber-rich diet levels and colon cancer.

Adapted from: Greenwald P, et al. *J Am Diet Assoc.* 1987;87:1178-1188.

12

Chemoprevention is the attempt to arrest or reverse premalignant cells during their progress to invasive malignancy using nontoxic physiologic mechanisms. Several classes of chemopreventive agents are under study:

- Carcinogen-blocking agents:
  - Oltipraz: enhances the detoxication of carcinogen
  - Indole-3-carbinol: inhibits the metabolic activation of procarcinogens
- Promotion suppressors:
  - Ornithine decarboxylase inhibitors: difluoromethylornithine (DFMO)
  - Cyclooxygenase type 2 inhibitor such as aspirin and sulindac (**Table 12.5 and Figure 12.14**)
  - Apoptosis-inducer like sulindac-sulfone
- Antioxidants:
  - Betacarotene
  - Vitamin E
  - Curcumin.

Surrogate endpoint biomarkers consist of intermediate biomarkers of carcinogenesis or biochemical markers of tumor progression (**Table 12.6**):

- Adenomatous polyps and/or aberrant crypt development
- Dysplasia indices such as nuclear antigens, PCNA, or KI-67
- Genomic indicators such as micronuclei, DNA ploidy, p53, apoptosis assay.

Recent basic scientific information suggests that a new strategy for preventing CRC may be possible utilizing cyclooxygenase 2 (Cox-2) inhibitors (**Table 12.5**). Cox-2 is overexpressed in tumors and causes increased prostaglandin synthesis, which contributes

TABLE 12.5 — COX-2 AND CHEMOPREVENTION

Cox-2 and CRC
- Overexpression of the gene for Cox-2 ↑ prostaglandin synthesis →↑ tumors
- Min mice lack APC →↑ polyps with ↑ Cox-2 especially in bowel stroma
- Double mutant mice for APC and Cox-2 have few polyps
- ↑ Cox-2 activity suppresses apoptosis
- Cox-2 regulates CRC-induced angiogenesis

Cox-2 Inhibitors and Chemoprevention
- Nonsteroidal anti-inflammatory drugs inhibit both Cox-1 and Cox-2, which can result in gastrointestinal ulceration and bleeding
- Sulindac decreases adenomas in FAP patients
- Selective Cox-2 inhibitor (MF-tricyclic) decreases polyps in APC-defective mice
- Phase I/II studies of MF-tricyclic are pending

Abbreviations: Cox, cyclooxygenase; CRC, colorectal cancer; APC, adenomatous polyposis coli [gene] (gene mutated in FAP); FAP, familial adenomatous polyposis.

FIGURE 12.14 — SULINDAC METABOLISM

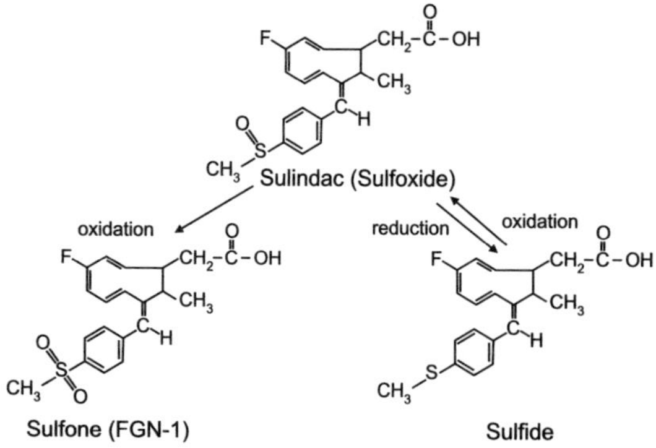

Adapted from: Duggan DE, et al. *Clin Pharmacol Ther.* 1977;21:326-335.

TABLE 12.6 — FGN-1 (EXISULIND) IN FAMILIAL ADENOMATOUS POLYPOSIS RECTAL POLYPS: PHASE I/II TRIAL

- Polyp regression in 89% of patients — polyps became flat, developed "halo"
- >50% increase in apoptosis, no change in Ki67
- Both number of polyps detected and median size of polyps stabilized or decreased with chronic exposure

Adapted from: Van Stalk R, et al. *Gastroenterology.* 1998;114: 696a.

to tumor growth. In a mouse model, which lacks the adenomatous polyposis coli (APC) gene, polyps spontaneously develop in the small and large intestine. These polyps contain greatly increased levels of cyclooxygenase. Double-mutant mice that lack both APC and Cox-2 have few polyps, suggesting that there is an interaction between the APC gene and the gene responsible for Cox-2 production. Animal and tissue culture research indicates that the Cox-2 activity suppresses apoptosis or programmed cell death and also regulates the angiogenesis in CRC.

Nonsteroidal anti-inflammatory drugs (NSAIDs) inhibit both cyclooxygenase 1 (Cox-1) and Cox-2; Cox-1 protects the intestine from acid-induced ulceration and bleeding. Sulindac, a long-acting NSAID, decreases polyp formation in patients with familial adenomatous polyposis (FAP) through the mechanism of Cox-2 inhibition. However, the drug has considerable side effects due to gastrointestinal ulceration and bleeding. Sulindac is metabolized (**Figure 12.14**) to a sulfide, which is an effective anti-inflammatory agent but inhibits both Cox-1 and Cox-2. Sulindac is also oxidized irreversibly to the sulindac-sulfone (FGN-1) which has no Cox-1 or Cox-2 inhibition but enhances apoptosis. The selective Cox-2 inhibitor MF-tricyclic decreases polyps in APC-defective mice, and sulindac-sulfone is effective in decreasing rectal polyps in patients with FAP (**Table 12.6**)

Six months of twice-daily treatment with 400 mg celecoxib in patients with FAP was associated with a 30% reduction in number and size of polyps.

To date, there are no chemopreventive agents that are suitable for routine use in CRC for which a randomized, placebo-controlled study has been completed.

SUGGESTED READINGS

Baron JA, Beach M, Mandel JS, et al. Calcium supplements for the prevention of colorectal adenomas. *N Engl J Med.* 1999;340:101-107.

Baron JA, Cole BF, Sandler RS, et al. A randomized trial of aspirin to prevent colorectal adenomas. *N Engl J Med.* 2003;348:891-899.

Duggan DE, Hare LE, Ditzler CA, Lei BW, Kwan KC. The disposition of sulindac. *Clin Pharmacol Ther.* 1977;21:326-335.

Engstrom PF, Benson AB, Saltz L. Colon cancer clinical practice guidelines in oncology. *J Nat Comp Cancer Network.* 2003;1:40-53.

Engstrom PF, Benson AB, Saltz L. Rectal cancer: clinical practice guidelines in oncology. *J Nat Comp Cancer Network.* 2003;1:54-63.

Greenwald P, Lanza E, Eddy GA. Dietary fiber in the reduction of colon cancer risk. *J Am Diet Assoc.* 1987;87:1178-1188.

Menko FH, Wijnen JT, Khan PM, Vasen HF, Oosterwijk MH. Genetic counseling in hereditary nonpolyposis colorectal cancer. *Oncology.* 1996;10:71-82.

O'Brien MJ, O'Keane JC, Zauber A, Gottlieb LS, Winawer SJ. Precursors of colorectal carcinoma. Biopsy and biologic markers. *Cancer.* 1992;70(suppl 5):1317-1327.

12

O'Brien MJ, Winawer SJ, Zauber AG, et al. The National Polyp Study. Patient and polyp characteristics associated with high-grade dysplasia in colorectal adenomas. *Gastroenterology.* 1990;98:371-379.

Potter JD. Reconciling the epidemiology, physiology, and molecular biology of colon cancer. *JAMA.* 1992;268:1573-1577.

Ries LA, Miller BA, Hanbey BF, et al. SEER Cancer Statistic Review, 1973-1991. Bethesda, Md: National Cancer Institute; 1994. NIH publication #94-2789.

Steinbach G, Lynch PM, Phillips RK, et al. The effect of celecoxib, a cyclooxygenase-2 inhibitor, in familial adenomatous polyposis. *N Engl J Med.* 2000;342:1946-1952.

Van Stalk R, Budd GT, Kresty R, et al. Effect of sulindac-sulfone on proliferation, apoptosis, and polyps in a clinical trial and familial adenomatous polyposis (FAP) with rectal polyps. *Gastroenterology.* 1998;114:696a.

Vargas PA, Alberts DS. Primary prevention of colorectal cancer through dietary modification. *Cancer.* 1992;70(suppl 5):1229-1235.

Vogelstein B, Fearon ER, Hamilton SR, et al. Genetic alterations during colorectal-tumor development. *N Engl J Med.* 1988;319:525-532.

Winawer SJ, Enker WE, Levin B. Colorectal cancer. In: Winawaer SJ, ed. *Management of Gastrointestinal Diseases.* New York, NY: Gower Medical; 1992.

Winawer SJ, Fletcher RH, Miller L, et al. Colorectal cancer screening: clinical guidelines and rationale. *Gastroenterology.* 1997;112:594-642.

13 Colorectal Cancer Screening

Normal-Risk Individuals

Screening studies should be performed in normal-risk individuals. They include:

- Annual fecal occult blood test (FOBT)
- Flexible sigmoidoscopy every 5 years
- Colonoscopy every 10 years
- Double-contrast barium enema (DCBE) every 5 to 10 years.

■ Fecal Occult Blood Test

The FOBT should be performed annually in normal-risk individuals. Two samples from each of three consecutive stool specimens (not by a digital rectal) should be examined. Dietary restriction should exist for 2 days, and the patient should be informed to avoid red meat, turnips, horseradish, salicylate, and vitamin C (**Table 13.1**). The guaiac-based method is recommended vs the immunochemical techniques (ie, Hemoccult II, Hemoccult II sensa).

A physician or his medical office should coordinate testing and proper interpretation of the FOBT to ensure compliance. Hemoccult sensitivity for detecting cancer is 72% to 78%, with a specificity of 98%. The positive predictive value for cancer is 10% to 17%. Thus, for every case of cancer detected, six to 10 patients need to undergo colonoscopy or barium enema as a result of a positive occult blood slide.

The Minnesota Trial randomized 46,551 people aged 50 to 80 years to annual FOBT screening, every-2-year FOBT screening or usual care (**Table 13.2**).

TABLE 13.1 — FACTORS AFFECTING FECAL OCCULT BLOOD TEST*

Avoid	Examples	False Positive	False Negative
Heme	Rare red meat	+	
Peroxidase activity	Turnips, horseradish	+	
Salicylates		+	
Vitamin C			+

* Ingestion of fiber (ie, fruits, vegetables) increases stool transit time and may avoid false-negative test results. Begin 24 hours before and continue through time of stool collection.

Adapted from: Winawer SJ, et al. *Gastroenterology*. 1997;112:594-642.

The 13-year cumulative mortality per 1000 from colorectal cancer was 5.88 in the annually screened group, 8.33 in the biannually screened group, and 8.83 in the control group. There was a 33% reduction in the group offered annual screening.

The Nottingham Study randomized 150,251 patients, 45 to 74 years of age and registered with general practitioners, to FOBT every 2 years or to receive usual care (**Table 13.3**). After a 7.8 years follow-up, there was a 15% reduction in mortality in the screened group.

The Danish Trial randomized 61,993 people aged 45 to 75 years to FOBT every 2 years vs usual care. After 10 years, there was an 18% reduction in colorectal cancer (CRC) mortality in the screened group.

In all of the studies noted above, colonoscopy was used to evaluate the patient with a positive FOBT. Alternative evaluation includes flexible sigmoidoscopy plus DCBE (**Table 13.4**).

■ **Flexible Sigmoidoscopy**

In normal risk individuals, a flexible sigmoidoscopy should be performed every 5 years. Flexible scopes identify nearly all cancers and polyps >1 cm and 70% to 85% of small polyps. It is estimated that a 60-cm scope can detect 40% to 60% of polyps and CRC while a 35-cm scope can detect 30% to 40% of lesions.

Three case-control studies show that rigid sigmoidoscopy was associated with 60% to 80% reduction in mortality from rectosigmoid carcinoma in patients with one or more studies in their lifetime. Patients with abnormalities on flexible sigmoidoscopy require full colonoscopy.

13

TABLE 13.2 — MINNESOTA COLORECTAL CANCER SCREENING STUDY*

| | Outcome by Study Group After 13 Years | | |
	Annual	Biennial	Control
CRC cases Incidence[†]	323 23	323 23	356 26
CRC deaths Mortality[†]	82 5.88	117 8.33	121 8.83
Mortality ratio	0.67	0.94	1.00

Cancers by Study Group and Duke's Classification

	Annual	Biennial	Control	5-Year Survival (%)
A	107	98	88	94.3
B	101	95	120	84.4
C	80	100	82	56.6
D	33	41	65	2.4
All	354	368	394	70.0

Abbreviations: CRC, colorectal cancer.

* 46,551 people 50 to 80 years, randomized.
† Per 1000.

Adapted from: Mandel JS, et al. *N Engl J Med.* 1993;328:1365-1371.

13

TABLE 13.3 — NOTTINGHAM FECAL OCCULT BLOOD TEST SCREENING STUDY

Cancer Stage Test vs Control (%)			
Duke's Classification	Tested (n = 76)	Not Tested (n = 81)	Control (n = 121)
A	53*	12	11
B	26	27	33
C	17	20	33
D	4*	31	22

	Screening Cycle		
	1st	2nd	3rd
+ FOBT (%)	2.3	1.7	0.3
Neoplasm (#/1000)	10.3	5.3	1.6
Interval cancers		20 (22%)	

Abbreviations: FOBT, fecal occult blood test.

* $p < 0.001$.

Adapted from: Hardcastle JD, et al. *Lancet.* 1996;348:1472-1477.

TABLE 13.4 — SUMMARY OF THE CHARACTERISTICS OF COLORECTAL CANCER SCREENING TESTS

Screening Test	Overall Performance	Complexity	Potential Effectiveness	Evidence Effectiveness	Screening Test Risk
FOBT	Intermediate for cancers, low for polyps	Lowest	Lowest	Strongest	Lowest
Flexible sigmoidoscopy	High for up to half of the colon	Intermediate	Intermediate	Intermediate	Intermediate
FOBT + flexible sigmoidoscopy	Same as flexible sigmoidoscopy and FOBT	Intermediate	Intermediate	Intermediate	Intermediate
DCBE	High	High	High	Weakest	Intermediate
Colonoscopy	Highest	Highest	Highest	Weakest	Highest

Abbreviations: FOBT, fecal occult blood test; DCBE, double-contrast barium enema.

Note: The costs of the screening tests themselves, also an important characteristic, vary, but the costs of the screening strategies, lifetime programs of screening, and follow-up of abnormal test result(s) are comparable. Complexity involves patient preparation, inconvenience, facilities and equipment needed, and patient discomfort.

Adapted from: Winawer SJ, et al. *Gastroenterology.* 1997;112:594-642.

13

■ **Colonoscopy**

Colonoscopy is considered the gold standard, with a sensitivity of 97% for cancer and a specificity of 100% for polyps or cancer. It should be performed every 10 years in normal-risk individuals. There is indirect evidence that people who have undergone colonoscopy or polypectomy have a 40% to 50% reduction in colorectal cancer incidence. Colonoscopy is recommended only for surveillance of patients with personal history of polyps or CRC or a family history of familial adenomatous polyposis (FAP) or hereditary nonpolyposis colon cancer (HNPCC).

■ **Double-Contrast Barium Enema**

A DCBE should be performed in normal-risk individuals every 5 to 10 years. There are no studies evaluating screening with DCBE alone as a means to reduce the incidence and mortality of CRC. It may be used for follow-up of abnormal findings (adenomatous polyp >1 cm or carcinoma) in patients:

- Whose large (>1-cm diameter) or multiple adenomatous polyps are found and removed at colonoscopy; they should have an examination of the colon repeated in 3 years
- Who have had a normal colonoscopy or a single, small tubular adenoma; they should have an examination within 5 years
- With invasive cancer, large sessile polyps or numerous adenomas; they should be individualized with more frequent (ie, 6-month to 1-year) repeat colonoscopy.

■ **Summary**

Table 13.4 compares the characteristics of the available CRC screening tests. Colonoscopy is the most accurate and highly effective method for screening for CRC. However, it has the highest complexity and the highest risk for inadvertent complications; evidence for effectiveness in the population setting is weak. On the other hand, the FOBT has the lowest complexity, the strongest evidence for reducing mortality in a randomized controlled trial setting and the lowest risk for side effects but also low effectiveness or efficiency. Combining FOBT and flexible sigmoidoscopy provides high performance plus intermediate complexity, risk, and potential effectiveness.

Positive Family History With Colon Cancer or Adenomatous Polyp

Figure 13.1 presents an algorithm for CRC screening and surveillance in average-risk and increased-risk populations. The following is additional information that should be considered by the clinician when faced with a decision to provide office surveillance for CRC.

Colorectal cancer is more common in patients with a positive family history (sibling, parent, child) of polyp or CRC (excluding HNPCC, FAP), particularly in individuals with one or more first-degree relatives with CRC or adenomatous polyp. Cancers generally appear at a younger age or age younger than 50 years. In such patients, screening for colorectal neoplasia should begin at age 40 years, utilizing FOBT, and perhaps flexible sigmoidoscopy (see normal- or average-risk screening above).

A history suggestive of HNPCC requires:
- Extended pedigree analysis of:
  - Colon cancer in primary and secondary family members
  - Colon cancer at age <50 years
  - Multiple generations affected
  - Right-sided colon cancer
  - Multiple primary sites, including colon, endometrium, ureteral, small bowel, stomach

13

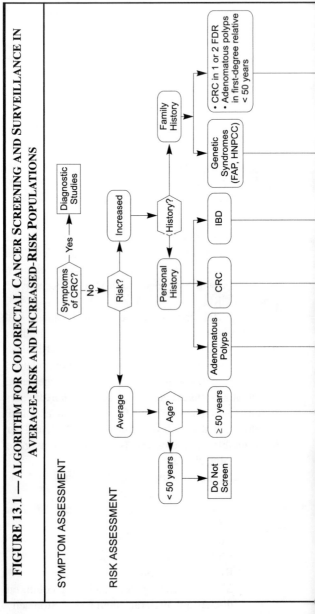

FIGURE 13.1 — ALGORITHM FOR COLORECTAL CANCER SCREENING AND SURVEILLANCE IN AVERAGE-RISK AND INCREASED-RISK POPULATIONS

SYMPTOM ASSESSMENT

- Symptoms of CRC? — Yes → Diagnostic Studies
- No

RISK ASSESSMENT

Risk?

- Average → Age?
  - < 50 years → Do Not Screen
  - ≥ 50 years
- Increased → History?
  - Personal History
    - Adenomatous Polyps
    - CRC
    - IBD
  - Family History
    - Genetic Syndromes (FAP, HNPCC)
    - CRC in 1 or 2 FDR
    - Adenomatous polyps in first-degree relative < 50 years

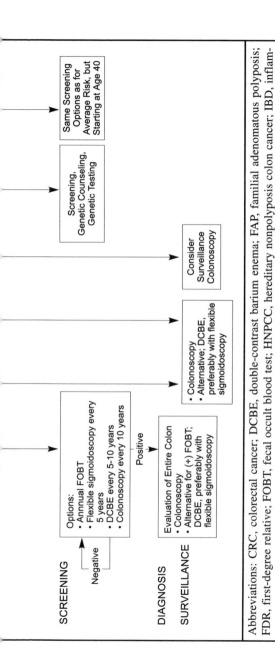

SCREENING

Negative

Options:
• Annual FOBT
• Flexible sigmoidoscopy every 5 years
• DCBE every 5-10 years
• Colonoscopy every 10 years

Positive

→ Colonoscopy
• Alternative; DCBE, preferably with flexible sigmoidoscopy

Screening, Genetic Counseling, Genetic Testing

Same Screening Options as for Average Risk, but Starting at Age 40

DIAGNOSIS

Evaluation of Entire Colon
• Colonoscopy
• Alternative for (+) FOBT, DCBE, preferably with flexible sigmoidoscopy

SURVEILLANCE

→ Consider Surveillance Colonoscopy

Abbreviations: CRC, colorectal cancer; DCBE, double-contrast barium enema; FAP, familial adenomatous polyposis; FDR, first-degree relative; FOBT, fecal occult blood test; HNPCC, hereditary nonpolyposis colon cancer; IBD, inflammatory bowel disease.

Adapted from: Winawer SJ, et al. *Gastroenterology.* 1997;112:594-642.

13

- Genetic counseling/testing of eligible family members:
  - Obtain a family history that includes parents, siblings, offspring, uncles, grandparents, and additional relatives with cancer
  - Minimal data obtained from each relative should include:
    - Current age and age at diagnosis of cancer
    - Date/age and cause of death
    - Type of cancer, noting multiple primaries
    - Other inherited conditions
    - Ethnicity/country of origin
    - Suspected colon cancer syndromes (ie, Muir-Torre, Turcot, Peutz-Jeghers)
  - Educate patients about recessive genetic inheritance and variable or delayed penetrance, multiple cancer primary sites
  - Counsel patient about genetic testing, cost, and usefulness
- If HPNCC is suspected, and tumors from affected family members are available for testing:
  - Test for replication error phenotype (RER) (microsatellite instability) in cancer
  - If RER positive, consider genetic mutation testing for hMSH-2 or hMLH-1 after appropriate genetic counseling
- Consider colonoscopy at age 20 to 25 years; repeat every 1 to 2 years
- For women, consider transvaginal ultrasound or endometrial aspirate annually beginning at age 25 to 35
- If patient has adenoma or adenocarcinoma, consider subtotal colectomy with ileorectal anastomosis or proctocolectomy if rectal cancer exists. Consider total abdominal hysterectomy/bilateral salpingo-oophorectomy at the time of colon surgery.

If a history of FAP exists and the patient has a personal history of FAP, a colectomy is required by age 25 years to reduce the likelihood of invasive cancer. Following postcolectomy with ileoproctostomy, the patient should undergo sigmoidoscopy every 6 months for 3 years, upper endoscopy every 4 years, and physical examination every 1 to 2 years. Patients with FAP postcolectomy may benefit from sulindac or sulindac-sulfone to reduce polyp formation in the rectum.

Presymptomatic individuals with a positive history of FAP should be considered for adenomatous polyposis coli (APC) genetic testing. The APC-positive individual should have flexible sigmoidoscopy every 12 months, beginning at puberty. If polyps are discovered, follow management above for personal history of FAP. The APC-negative individual should have flexible sigmoidoscopy once at age 25 and then routine screening beginning at age 50. Nontested individuals should have flexible sigmoidoscopy every 12 months until age 24, every 2 years until 34, every 3 years until 44, and every 3 to 5 years thereafter.

Patients with inflammatory bowel disease are at increased risk for colon cancer, depending on duration and extent of disease; colectomy can eliminate the risk of cancer. Therefore, it is common practice to perform surveillance colonoscopy every 1 to 2 years, beginning after 8 years if pancolitis or after 15 years in those with colitis involving only the left colon.

13

SUGGESTED READINGS

Hardcastle JD, Chamberlain JO, Robinson MH, et al. Randomised controlled trial of faecal-occult-blood screening for colorectal cancer. *Lancet.* 1996;348:1472-1477.

Lieberman DA, Weiss DG, Bond JH, Ahnen DJ, Garewal H, Chejfec G. Use of colonoscopy to screen asymptomatic adults for colorectal cancer. *N Engl J Med.* 2000;343:162-168.

Mandel JS, Bond JH, Church TR, et al. Reducing mortality from colorectal cancer by screening for fecal occult blood. Minnesota Colon Cancer Control Study. *N Engl J Med.* 1993;328:1365-1371.

Winawer SJ, Fletcher RH, Miller L, et al. Colorectal cancer screening: clinical guidelines and rationale. *Gastroenterology.* 1997;112:594-642.

Winawer SJ, Stewart ET, Zauber AG, et al. A comparison of colonoscopy and double-contrast barium enema for surveillance after polypectomy. *N Engl J Med.* 2000;342:1766-1772.

14 Management of Colorectal Cancer

Staging Colorectal Cancer

The staging criteria are dependent upon the pathologic examination of a completely resected colon or rectal cancer. The American Joint Commission on Cancer (AJCC) Staging System, which stipulates primary tumor, nodal involvement, and distant metastasis (TNM), has replaced the Duke's classification or its Astler-Coller modification. Staging is based on the natural history of the tumor, which usually starts as a polyp with *in situ* carcinoma and invades the wall of the bowel. **Figure 14.1** shows a cross-sectional view of the large bowel; it indicates the successive layers from the lumen to the peritoneal cavity which correspond to the progressive T stage or Duke stage. Thus, a stage II T3 (B2) tumor invades through the muscularis propria into the subserosa but not through the serosa to the visceral peritoneum. Metastasis may involve regional lymph nodes or spread by the blood stream to distant organs (ie, liver, lung, bone, and brain). **Table 14.1** describes the stage classification by pathologic description and compares the AJCC TNM stage to the Astler-Coller modification of the Duke stage.

Because the prognosis deteriorates with advancing stage, management of colorectal cancer (CRC) is based on the stage of the disease and performance status of the patient. **Figure 14.2** shows the disease-free survival according to the surgical stage of colon cancer based on gastrointestinal tumor study group data and utilizing the Astler-Coller classification. **Figure 14.3** shows rectal cancer disease-free survival based

FIGURE 14.1 — ANATOMIC HISTOLOGY
OF THE LARGE BOWEL

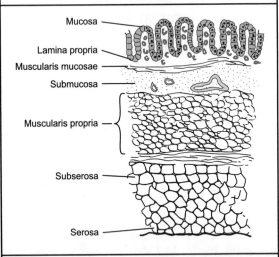

Mucosa
Lamina propria
Muscularis mucosae
Submucosa
Muscularis propria
Subserosa
Serosa

Layers are identified from the lumen (top) to the peritoneal cavity (bottom).

on the Astler-Coller classification. In both sets of data, patients who have tumors that are limited to the bowel wall and have not spread to the serosa or to regional lymph nodes have a significantly better survival than stage III (C1 or C2) patients.

Clinical Symptoms

Colorectal cancer clinical symptoms (**Table 14.2**) include:

- Cancer of the right or ascending colon:
  - Obstruction is late in the course and is usually due to lesions near the ileocecal valve
  - Pain is ill-defined and located in right midabdomen

- Bleeding is usually occult, but when acute, it produces a brick-red stool
- Weakness due to chronic anemia is common
- Cancer of left or descending colon:
  - Obstruction is common and produces change in caliber of the stool
  - Pain is usually colicky and made worse by ingestion of food
  - Bleeding is usually intermittent and may be occult or result in red blood mixed with stool
  - Weakness due to anemia is infrequent
- Cancer of the rectum:
  - Obstruction is rare and late in the course of the disease
  - Pain is steady, gnawing; tenesmus is caused by tumor infiltration of perisphincteric lymphatic vessels
  - Bleeding is usually bright red, coating stool, and all too often mistaken for hemorrhoidal bleeding
  - Weakness due to anemia is rare.

Principles of Surgical Treatment

Adenomatous polyps with *in situ* low-grade adenocarcinoma (superficial carcinoma without deep invasion of stock of polyp) can be treated with polypectomy only if the margin indicates all cancer was completely resected. Invasive colon carcinoma, villous adenoma, or villoglandular adenoma with cancer, which is fragmented or has positive margins, requires colectomy with *en bloc* removal of regional lymph nodes. *En bloc* removal of regional lymph nodes is necessary to facilitate pathologic review of pericolonic and perirectal soft tissue and analysis of pericolonic or perirectal lymphatic tissue. Surgical visualization, palpation and, where appropriate, intraoperative ultra-

14

TABLE 14.1 — COLORECTAL CANCER: STAGE CLASSIFICATION AND GROUPING

Pathological Description	AJCC (1992; 4th Edition)	Astler-Coller Modification of Duke's Classification
Carcinoma *in situ*	Stage 0 – T1, N0, M0	Stage 0
Tumor invades submucosa	Stage I – T1, N0, M0	Stage I – A
Tumor invades muscularis propria	Stage I – T2, N0, M0	Stage I – B1
Tumor invades through muscularis propria into subserosa or nonperitonealized perirectal tissue	Stage II – T3, N0, M0	Stage II – B2
Tumor directly invades other organs or strictures and/or perforates visceral peritoneum	Stage II – T4, N0, M0	Stage II – B3
Any degree of bowel-wall invasion with regional node metastasis, without distant metastasis	Stage IIIA – Any T, N1, M0 (1-3 nodes) Stage IIIB – Any T, N2, M0 (>4 nodes)	Stage III – C1, C2

| Any degree of bowel-wall invasion with or without nodal metastasis but with any distant metastasis | Stage IV – Any T, any N, M1 | Stage IV – D |

Abbreviations: AJCC, American Joint Commission on Cancer.

Adapted from: Green FL, ed. *AJCC Cancer Staging Manual*. 6th ed. New York: Springer Verlag; 2002:113-123.

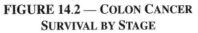

FIGURE 14.2 — COLON CANCER SURVIVAL BY STAGE

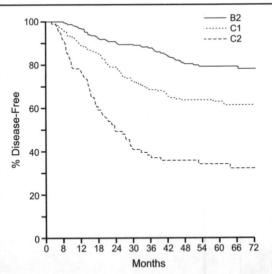

Probability of disease-free survival according to surgical stage of colon cancer – GITSG modification of Astler-Coller classification.

Adapted from: Gastrointestinal Tumor Study Group. *N Engl J Med*. 1985;312:1465-1472.

sonographic evaluation of adjacent or noncontiguous target organs for distant spread is mandatory (**Figure 14.4**).

Laparoscopic-assisted colon resection should be limited to patients with either far-advanced distant disease, significant comorbid illness or in highly formalized multi-institutional clinical trials. Functional consequences of surgical resection should be minimized consistent with curative principles of surgery:

- Right hemicolectomy, transverse colectomy and left hemicolectomy are defined anatomically by

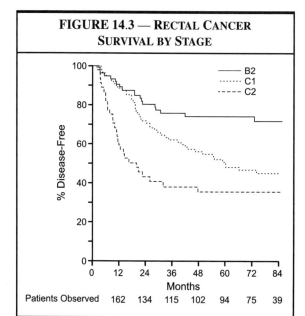

FIGURE 14.3 — RECTAL CANCER SURVIVAL BY STAGE

| Patients Observed | 162 | 134 | 115 | 102 | 94 | 75 | 39 |

Time to recurrence of rectal carcinoma according to disease stage of colon cancer – GITSG modification of Astler-Coller classification.

Adapted from: Gastrointestinal Tumor Study Group. *N Engl J Med.* 1985;312:1465-1472.

the ileocolic, the middle colic, and the right colic vessels.

- Patients with T1 and T2 adenocarcinoma of the mild and distal rectum may be cured with perianal, transanal, transcoccygeal, or transsacral approaches or low-end anterior approaches with coloanal reanastomoses, thereby avoiding abdominal peritoneal resection with descending colostomy.

Patients with stage III lesions are candidates for adjuvant chemotherapy and/or radiotherapy treatment.

TABLE 14.2 — VARIATION IN SYMPTOMS OF RIGHT COLON, LEFT COLON AND RECTAL CANCER

Symptom	Right Colon	Left Colon	Rectum
Pain	Ill-defined	Colicky*	Steady, gnawing
Obstruction	Infrequent†	Common	Infrequent
Bleeding	Brick red	Red, mixed with stool	Bright red, coating stool
Weakness‡	Common	Infrequent	Infrequent

* Made worse by the ingestion of food.
† If obstruction occurs, tumor often is located at ileocecal valve region.
‡ Weakness secondary to anemia.

Adapted from: Sugarbaker PH. In: Steele G Jr, et al, eds. *Colorectal Cancer: Current Concepts in Diagnosis and Treatment.* New York, NY: Marcel Dekker, Inc; 1986:59-98.

FIGURE 14.4 — ANATOMIC SEGMENTS, ARTERIAL AND VENOUS BLOOD SUPPLY AND SURGICAL RESECTIONS OF THE COLON AND RECTUM

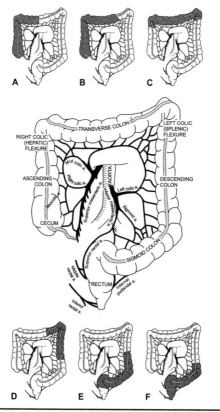

(A) Right hemicolectomy; (B) extended right hemocolectomy; (C) transverse colectomy; (D) left hemicolectomy; (E) sigmoid resection; (F) rectosigmoid resection.

Adapted from: Sugarbaker PH. In: *Colorectal Cancer: Current Concepts in Diagnosis and Treatment.* New York, NY: Marcel Dekker, Inc; 1986; and Jones T, Shepard WC. *A Manual of Surgical Anatomy.* Philadelphia, Pa: WB Saunders Co; 1945.

14

Principles of Radiotherapy Management of Colorectal Cancer

Because the pattern of failure after rectal cancer surgery is to local and regional lymph nodes, postoperative radiotherapy can significantly reduce pelvic recurrence. Radiation toxicity can be minimized by excluding small bowel from the pelvis (retroperitonealized pelvic floor), treating the patient prone with the bladder distended and using small doses per fraction.

Preoperative radiation may:

- Increase resectability
- Enhance effect because tissues are well vascularized and oxygenated
- Reduce toxicity because small bowel is freely mobile
- Theoretically, decrease implantation of viable cells during surgical manipulation.

Postoperative radiation avoids delay of surgery, is given after the extent of the disease is defined and thus spares patients with stage I and stage IV disease. Adjuvant radiotherapy significantly reduces nodal recurrence and local recurrence of rectal carcinoma, but this has not translated into increased overall 5-year survival.

Principles of Chemotherapy

The fluoropyrimidine, 5-fluorouracil (5-FU) is the mainstay for systemic chemotherapy of recurrent or metastatic CRC. The objective response rate to 5-FU and metastatic disease is 15% to 20% with only the responding patient showing a median survival of 12 to 18 months. Therapeutic effect can be enhanced by administering 5-FU by continuous infusion or by combining 5-FU with leucovorin.

Intrahepatic artery infusion of 5-FU or flurodeoxidurodine (FUDR) has been successfully used to palliate patients with liver metastasis from CRC. Irinotecan (Camptosar) is approved for the treatment of a patient with progressive metastatic disease that has failed 5-FU-based therapy. Patients with stage III colon cancer who are treated with 5-FU plus leucovorin or 5-FU plus levamisole have approximately a 20% improvement in disease-free survival compared with surgery alone (**Figures 14.5 and 14.6**).

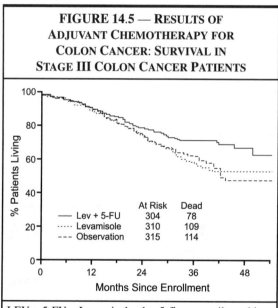

FIGURE 14.5 — RESULTS OF ADJUVANT CHEMOTHERAPY FOR COLON CANCER: SURVIVAL IN STAGE III COLON CANCER PATIENTS

	At Risk	Dead
Lev + 5-FU	304	78
Levamisole	310	109
Observation	315	114

LEV + 5-FU = Levamisole plus 5-fluorouracil combination therapy.

Adapted from: Moertel CG, et al. *N Engl J Med*. 1990;322:352-358.

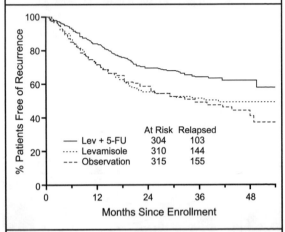

FIGURE 14.6 — RESULTS OF ADJUVANT CHEMOTHERAPY FOR COLON CANCER: RECURRENCE-FREE INTERVAL IN STAGE III COLON CANCER PATIENTS

	At Risk	Relapsed
Lev + 5-FU	304	103
Levamisole	310	144
Observation	315	155

LEV + 5-FU = Levamisole plus 5-fluorouracil combination therapy.

Adapted from: Moertel CG, et al. *N Engl J Med*. 1990;322:352-358.

Management Guidelines for Colon Cancer

The initial workup for the management of colon cancer should include:

- History:
  - Weight loss
  - Anemia
  - Obstruction symptoms
  - Change in bowel size and frequency
  - Blood loss
  - Careful family history of bowel cancer
- Physical examination:

- Rectal exam for mass or blood
- Adenopathy in the neck
- Palpable or enlarged liver
- Abdominal mass
• Full colonoscopy or flexible sigmoidoscopy and double-contrast barium enema (DCBE)
• Complete blood count (CBC):
  - Platelets
  - Liver function studies
  - Carcinoembryonic antigen (CEA)
• Chest film and posteroanterior (PA) lateral
• Computed tomography (CT) scan; abdomen and pelvis if clinically indicated (especially obstructing or large invasive colonic tumors).

The initial treatment is based on the clinical findings. If an adenomatous polyp or villous adenoma with cancer at polypectomy is found, a full colonoscopy should be performed if not already accomplished. A pathologic review is necessary if the superficial lesion was completely resected; no further surgery is required. If there is a deep invasion or fragmented removal of colectomy, an *en bloc* resection of regional lymph nodes should be accomplished.

If an ulcerated mass or invasive carcinoma is discovered on endoscopic biopsy, colectomy with *en bloc* removal of regional lymph nodes is indicated. If there is an obstructing or perforated lesion which is resectable, a colectomy with *en bloc* removal of regional lymph nodes should be performed. If the obstructing or perforated lesion is in an unprepared bowel, consider diverting colostomy with later palliative resection, if possible. If colon cancer with suspected or biopsied distant metastasis is found, consider palliative resection of primary tumor; a solitary liver metastasis can be resected at laparotomy.

14

Adjuvant chemotherapy depends on stage at diagnosis:

- Stage 0 or stage I (T1-2N0M0): no adjuvant therapy is required following definitive resection
- Stage II (T3N0M0): adjuvant 5-FU/leucovorin for 6 months if lesion caused obstruction or perforation. There is no evidence that patients with uncomplicated stage II colon cancer benefit from adjuvant chemotherapy
- Stage III (T1-4N1M0): adjuvant chemotherapy using 5-FU plus levamisole for 12 months or 5-FU plus leucovorin for 6 months is required
- Stage IV (T1-4N0-1M1):
  - If one to three small liver metastases, consider resection followed by adjuvant 5-FU/leucovorin chemotherapy
  - If multiple unresectable liver metastasis and primary bowel is resected, consider intrahepatic artery infusional therapy using FUDR
  - If unresectable abdominal metastasis or lung metastasis, consider systemic therapy with 5-FU/leucovorin
  - Clinical trial or observation may be appropriate in patients presenting with stage IV disease.

Monitoring and follow-up surveillance after definitive management of stage 0, I, II, or III cancers includes:

- Physical examination, including digital rectal exam and stool for fecal occult blood test (FOBT), every 3 months for 2 years, then every 6 months for 5 years, then annually
- Colonoscopy at 1 year; repeat in 1 year if abnormal or every 3 to 5 years if examination was normal
- The use of CEA as a follow-up test should be considered if it was elevated prior to surgery and if the patient is a candidate for aggressive

resection of metastatic lesions; CEA in this situation should be repeated every 2 to 3 months for 2 years
- The use of CBC, liver function studies, chest film and CT scan depends on the patient's clinical condition.

The management of patients with recurrent or metastatic colon cancer should include:
- Consideration of surgical resection in patients with isolated recurrences (liver, lung, or ovaries)
- In patients with widespread recurrence, consider palliative chemotherapy:
  - If no prior chemotherapy, then 5-FU plus leucovorin
  - If progressed after adjuvant or bolus 5-FU-based therapy, consider infusional 5-FU or infusional 5-FU/leucovorin or irinotecan
- In patients with obstruction, consider percutaneous gastrostomy or bypass surgery
- In patients with bone metastasis, consider palliative radiotherapy
- In unresectable patients, consider observation or hospice care.

Colon cancer chemotherapy regimens include:
- Adjuvant 5-FU/leucovorin 5-days, 5-FU 425 mg/m^2, intravenous bolus (IVB) days 1 through 5, leucovorin 20 mg/m^2 IVB days 1 through 5, repeat both every 28 days for 6 cycles
- Adjuvant 5-FU/leucovorin (weekly high dose) 5-FU 500 mg/m^2 IVB days 1, 8, 15, 22, 29, 36; leucovorin 500 mg/m^2 IVB days 1, 8, 15, 22, 29, 36; repeat every 8 weeks
- Adjuvant 5-FU/leucovorin (weekly low dose) 5-FU 500 mg/m^2 IVB days 1, 8, 15, 22, 29, 36; leucovorin 20 mg/m^2 IVB days 1, 8, 15, 22, 29, 36; repeat every 8 weeks

14

- 5-FU/leucovorin/irinotecan (Saltz) x 4 every 6 week cycle:
  - Irinotecan 125 mg/m^2 every week
  - 5-FU 500 mg/m^2 every week
  - Leucovorin 20 mg/m^2 every week
- 5-FU/leucovorin/irinotecan (Folfiri) 2 week cycle:
  - Irinotecan 180 mg/m^2 day 1 every 2 weeks
  - Leucovorin 200 mg/m^2 day 1 every 2 weeks
  - 5-FU 400 mg/m^2 day 1 every 2 weeks
  - 5-FU 2.4-3.0 gm/m^2 over 46 hours day 1 every 2 weeks
- 5-FU/leucovorin/oxaliplatin (Folfox) 2 week cycle:
  - Oxaliplatin 85-130 mg/m^2 day 1 every 2 week
  - Leucovorin 200 mg/m^2 day 1 every 2 weeks
  - 5-FU 400 mg/m^2 bolus day 1 every 2 weeks
  - 5-FU 2.4 gm/m^2 over 46 hours day 1 every 2 weeks
- Salvage irinotecan, irinotecan 125 mg/m^2 IV over 90 minutes days 1, 8, 15, 22; repeat every 6 weeks.

Management Guidelines for Rectal Cancer

For the initial workup for rectal cancer, see the guidelines for the workup of colon cancer. The initial treatment is based on the clinical findings. If a rectal polyp with carcinoma *in situ* is discovered, a polypectomy is sufficient.

For a rectal polyp <3 cm with invasion of stock or unclear margin, the options include:
- Full-thickness rectal resection by transanal or transcoccygeal route
- Endocavitary radiation can be considered for well-differentiated, exophytic lesion without ulceration or fixation

- Fulguration is an option only in highly selected cases because there is high risk of recurrence.

In patients with early-stage, invasive carcinoma >6 cm from the anal verge, low anterior resection with a 2-cm to 3-cm distal margin is recommended. In patients with early-stage (not fixed) invasive rectal carcinoma <5 cm from the anal verge, consider low anterior resection with coloanal anastomosis or an abdominal peritoneal (AP) resection.

In patients with rectal carcinoma with tumor adherence to or invasion of bladder or prostate, presacrum or pelvic sidewalls, consider preoperative chemotherapy/radiation to decrease tumor volume in order to allow AP resection followed by further radiation therapy and chemotherapy. Adjuvant therapy depends on stage at diagnosis:

- Stage 0 and stage I (T1, N0, M0): do not require chemotherapy or radiotherapy
- Poor-risk stage I (T1, N0, M0): treated with transanal resection should be considered for radiation with or without 5-FU-based chemotherapy
- Stage II or stage III rectal carcinoma: patients should receive radiotherapy plus 5-FU chemotherapy
- Stage IV: patients who have resectable liver, lung or ovarian metastasis should have definitive surgical therapy of the rectal tumor followed by 5-FU therapy plus pelvic radiotherapy
- Stage IV: patients who are not resectable for cure can be considered for colostomy and palliative pelvic radiotherapy or referred to hospice care.

14

5-FU radiotherapy postresection, adjuvant therapy involved 5-FU 500 IVB days 1 through 5 and 28 through 32, beginning 20 to 70 days postsurgery; radiotherapy 180 cGy/day, 5-days/week for 6 weeks (total 5040 cGy) beginning day 56; 5-FU 225 mg/m^2/day CIV throughout radiation period; 5-FU 400 mg/m^2/day IVB days 1 through 5, given 1 month after radiotherapy; 5-FU 500 mg/m^2/day IVB days 1 through 5 given 28 days after previous 5-FU course.

SUGGESTED READINGS

Gastrointestinal Tumor Study Group. Prolongation of the disease-free interval in surgically treated rectal carcinoma. *N Engl J Med.* 1985;312:1465-1472.

Green FL, ed. *AJCC Cancer Staging Manual.* 6th ed. New York: Springer Verlag; 2002:113-123.

Greenwald P, Kelloff GJ, Boone CW, McDonald SS. Genetic and cellular changes in colorectal cancer: proposed targets of chemopreventive agents. *Cancer Epidemiol Biomarkers Prev.* 1995;4:691-702.

Jones T, Shepard WC, eds. *A Manual of Surgical Anatomy.* Philadelphia, Pa: WB Saunders Co; 1945.

Moertel CG. Chemotherapy for colorectal cancer. *N Engl J Med.* 1994;330:1136-1142.

Moertel CG, Fleming TR, Macdonald JS, et al. Levamisole and fluorouracil for adjuvant therapy of resected colon carcinoma. *N Engl J Med.* 1990;322:352-358.

Mulcahy ME, Benson AB. New agents for colorectal cancer. *J Nat Comp Cancer Network.* 2003;1:125-136.

Sugarbaker PH. Clinical evaluation of symptomatic patients. In: Steele G, Osteen RT, Osteen D, eds. *Colorectal Cancer: Current Concepts in Diagnosis and Treatment.* New York, NY: Marcel Dekker, Inc; 1986:59-98.

Zaheer S, Pemberton JH, Farouk R, Dozois RR, Wolff BG, Ilstrup D. Surgical treatment of adenocarcinoma of the rectum. *Ann Surg.* 1998;227:800-811.

15 Educational Material and Resource Information

American Cancer Society (ACS)
Phone: 1-800-ACS-2345
Website: www.cancer.org

This site and the free phone line provide information to patients on cancer treatment, early detection, prevention, as well as information on a variety of services available to cancer patients and their families.

American College of Gastroenterology (ACG)
PO Box 3009
Alexandria, VA 22302
Phone: 703/820-7400
Fax: 703/931-4520
Website: www.acg.gi.org

The American College of Gastroenterology (ACG) hosts a website that includes general information about the ACG, a physician forum with information about meetings, courses, practice guidelines and available publications, and a gastrointestinal (GI) patient's health source, including patient education brochures. The GI patient's health source includes information on colorectal cancer, screening and prevention of colorectal cancer, inflammatory bowel disease, diverticular disease, and irritable bowel syndrome, among other topics.

American Gastroenterological Association (AGA)
Seventh Floor
4930 Del Ray Ave.
Bethesda, MD 20814
Phone: 301/654-2055
Fax: 301/652-3890
Website: www.gastro.org

Founded in 1897, the American Gastroenterological Association (AGA) is the oldest nonprofit speciality medical society in the country. Their website includes a digestive health resource center, a gastroenterologist locator service, a digestive health initiative and other web links to sites of interest.

American Society for Gastrointestinal Endoscopy (ASGE)
Suite 202
1520 Kensington Road
Oak Brook, IL 60523
Phone: 630/573-0600
Fax: 630-573-0691
Website: www.asge.org

The American Society for Gastrointestinal Endoscopy (ASGE) promotes the highest standards of training and practice for gastrointestinal endoscopy. Their mission is to be the foremost resource for education in this field.

American Society of Colon and Rectal Surgeons (ASCRS)
Suite 550
85 W. Algonquin Road
Arlington Heights, IL 60005
Phone: 847/290-9184
Fax: 847/290-9203
Website: www.fascrs.org/ascrs-home.html

The American Society of Colon and Rectal Surgeons (ASCRS) website has information to aid patients in locating a colon and rectal surgeon in their area. Additionally, an ASCRS Discussion Group is linked, as well as the ASCRS Newsletter.

CancerNet
Suite 3036A
6116 Executive Blvd., MSC8322
Bethesda, MD 20892-8322
Website: cancernet.nci.nih.gov

CancerNet includes a variety of sources to help meet cancer information needs such as selected information from PDQ (the National Cancer Institute's [NCI] comprehensive cancer database), including summaries on cancer treatment, screening, prevention and supportive care, and information on ongoing clinical trials; CancerLit, the NCI's bibliographic database; and fact sheets, news and other resources. This website has information with patients and the public, health professionals and basic researchers, as well as links to other useful cancer-related websites. It is updated monthly.

Colon Cancer Information Library
Website: www.meds.com/mol/colon/index.html

The Colon Cancer Information Center provides in-depth information on colon cancer, colorectal cancer and treatments. The colon cancer information is intended for use by both oncology professionals and patients in the United States. Included are clinical trial information, major online cancer resources, major cancer center list, news group lists, disease information, cancer organizations and current news on cancer.

Crohn's and Colitis Foundation of America (CCFA)
17th Floor
386 Park Avenue South
New York, NY 10016-8804
Phone: 212/685-3440
Toll-free: 800/932-2423
Fax: 212/779-4098
Website: www.ccfa.org

The Crohn's and Colitis Foundation of America (CCFA) hosts this website with a physician's resource room, news updates about IBD, a library and research database, bookstore, weekly features and links to other IBD-related websites.

15

Crohn's and Colitis Foundation of Canada (CCFC)
Suite 600
60 St. Clair Avenue Eat
Toronto, Ontario
Canada M4T 1N5
Phone: 416/920-5035 and
800/387-1479
Fax: 416/929-0364
Website: www.ccfc.ca/en/index.html

The Crohn's and Colitis Foundation of Canada (CCFC)
believes that a cure will be found for Crohn's disease and
ulcerative colitis. To realize this, the CCFC is commit-
ted to raising increasing funds for medical research. The
CCFC also believes it is important to make all individuals with inflammatory bowel disease (IBD) aware of the
Foundation and to educate these individuals, their families, health professionals and the general public about
these diseases. Their website includes information about
the CCFC, IBD fact information, a resource library and
links to other related websites.

Digestive Disease National Coalition
Suite 200
507 Capitol Court NE
Washington, DC 20003
Phone: 202/544-7497
Fax: 202/546-7105
Website: www.ddnc.org

This organization informs the public and the health care
community about digestive diseases. It also seeks federal
funding for research, education and training. Brochures
and newsletters are available.

IBD News Digest
5801 South Ellis
Chicago, IL 60637
Phone: 800/289-6333 or
773/702-1234

The University of Chicago publishes *IBD News Digest*
which highlights research and patient-care projects of
their IBD team. These articles will be of particular inter-

est to IBD patients who wish to learn more about how innovations in basic science and new clinical trials are being used to improve the treatment of ulcerative colitis and Crohn's disease.

National Cancer Institute Information Service
Phone: 1-800-4-CANCER
TTY: 1-800-332-8615
Website: www.cancer.gov/cancerinfo

The Cancer Information Service (CIS) is a nationwide network of 19 regional offices supported by the National Cancer Institute (NCI), the US Government's primary agency for cancer research. As the voice of the National Cancer Institute, the CIS serves the public through two programs: a toll-free telephone service and an outreach program. The CIS can provide unbiased information in understandable language about specific types of cancer, as well as information on state-of-the-art care and the availability of clinical trials.

National Cancer Institute (NCI)
National Institutes of Health (NIH)
Suite 3036A
6116 Executive Blvd., MSC8322
Bethesda, Maryland 20892-8322
Website: www.cancer.gov/cancerinfo

The NCI is a component of the NIH. The NCI coordinates the National Cancer Program, which conducts and supports research, training, health information dissemination, and other programs with respect to the cause, diagnosis, prevention and treatment of cancer, rehabilitation from cancer, and the continuing care of cancer patients and the families of cancer patients. Links to other pertinent sites are available.

National Institutes of Diabetes and
Digestive and Kidney Diseases (NIDDK)
National Institutes of Health (NIH)
9000 Rockville Pike
Bethesda, MD 20892
Phone: 301/496-4000
Website: www.cancer.gov/cancerinfo

15

This website has information on constipation, Crohn's disease, diverticulosis and diverticulitis, irritable bowel syndrome, ulcerative colitis and many other digestive diseases. Links to national organizations serving patients concerned about digestive diseases are listed as well as links to national organizations serving professionals concerned about digestive diseases.

Pediatric Crohn's and Colitis Association
PO Box 188
Newton, MA 02468
Phone: 617/489-5854

This association focuses on all aspects of pediatric and adolescent Crohn's disease and ulcerative colitis, including medical, nutritional, psychological and social factors. Activities include information sharing, educational forums, newsletters, a hospital outreach program and support of research.

Physician Data Query (PDQ)
Phone: 800/422-6237
Website: www.cancer.gov/cancerinfo

PDQ is the National Cancer Institute's comprehensive cancer information database. It is comprised of three main types of information. Full-text statements based on the published literature that reflect the current status of the treatment, supportive care, prevention, and screening of cancer, as well as information about selected anti-cancer drugs. These statements are written in two versions, one for health care professionals and one for patients and their families. Summaries of clinical trials are given. Directories of physicians and organizations that provide cancer care are available. Access to the Journal of the National Cancer Institute is available at this website.

Society for Surgery of the Alimentary Tract (SSAT)
900 Cummings Center, #221-U
Beverly, MA 01915
Phone: 978/927-8330
Fax: 978/524-8890
Website: www.ssat.com
The website of the SSAT provides information about diseases of the alimentary tract, *Journal of Gastrointestinal Surgery*, and patient care guidelines.

**Society of American Gastrointestinal
Endoscopic Surgeons (SAGES)**
Suite 3000
2716 Ocean Park Blvd.
Santa Monica, CA 90405
Phone: 310/314-2404
Fax: 310/314-2585
Website: www.sages.org/sages.html

The Society of American Gastrointestinal Endoscopic Surgeons is the leading professional society representing more than 3000 board certified surgeons who use endoscopy and laparoscopy as an integral part of their treatment of patients.

15

INDEX

16

16

16

269

16

16

16

16

16

16

16

16

16